The CDA™ Book

Keith W. Boone

The CDA™ Book

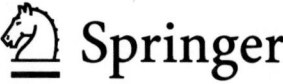 Springer

Author
Keith W. Boone
Norroway Ave 17
02368 Randolph
USA

ISBN 978-0-85729-335-0   e-ISBN 978-0-85729-336-7
DOI 10.1007/978-0-85729-336-7
Springer London Dordrecht Heidelberg New York

British Library Cataloguing in Publication Data
A catalogue record for this book is available from the British Library

Library of Congress Control Number: 2011922536

Cover design: eStudioCalamar, Figueres/Berlin

Printed on acid-free paper

Springer is part of Springer Science+Business Media (www.springer.com)

This book is dedicated to the memory William J. Boone,
Allen "Chris" Christman, Thomas Ross, and Josephine T. Ross,
and to my Mother, Gail Christman.

Preface

I've been meaning to write a book on CDA for at least 3 years. The first time I brought the idea up with possible collaborators, there seemed to be not enough time. There was simply too much work going on developing CDA implementation guides to carve out the time it would take. Those of us working on CDA implementation guides had very little time because our nights and weekends were often taken up by CDA based projects.

I started a blog in the middle of 2008 called Healthcare Standards where I write about the same almost daily. You can find it on the web at http://motorcycleguy.blogspot.com, or just follow me on twitter at @motorcycle_guy. The idea behind the blog was to have a place to publish information that I was constantly referring people to. There was some hope that I would be able to use material from the blog to help me create a book on CDA. Several parts of this book draw from material originally published on that blog.

The book came up again in a discussion with a standards colleague at the HL7 Working Group meeting in September of 2008 in Vancouver. She strongly encouraged me to write it, but again I demurred. We discussed it again about a year later in Atlanta and she finally convinced me that I could do it. If you happen to run into Kate Hamilton at an HL7 Working group meeting and enjoyed this book, thank her. Without her, this book might never have been written.

Writing began about a month later on November 14th of 2009, and nearly a year later the book is finished. The original working title was "The Little CDA™ Book", and I had hoped to have it finished by the end of summer. As you can see from the present title and text, it is no longer a little book.

Over the last seven years, I have been learning about CDA, and teaching what I have learned to others. In that process, I have learned a great deal about healthcare and electronic medical records. Quite of bit of that knowledge was freely shared with me by others, and the only way to pay back that kindness is to pay it forward to others.

You, my readers, are the recipients of that payment. You too can pay it forward by applying what you learn. My hope is that together we will create a healthcare system that can share meaningful information about patients their healthcare providers and with those patients who receive care.

Who This Book Is For

This book is for informatics students who want to learn about the HL7 CDA standard and software developers who need to implement it in healthcare information technology products. After reading this book you should know enough about CDA to make use of the CDA Implementation Guides described in the final chapter of this book, and to develop implementation guides on your own.

Prerequisites

This book is too short to cover everything you need to know to develop CDA implementations. You need to have at least a basic understanding of the following technologies to appreciate the content of this book.

Object-Oriented Design (OOD) – The CDA Specification and all HL7 Version 3 specifications use object oriented design principals. You will need to understand the ideas behind OOD including classes, associations, association classes and inheritance.

XML – The CDA Specification is built to use Extensible Markup Language (XML). This book does explain some of the more esoteric topics in that standard, but is not a substitute for experience or training in that standard.

Namespaces for XML – CDA requires the use of namespaces to describe the format of a clinical document. You will need to understand how namespaces work in XML to use this book.

XSLT – XSLT is often used to display CDA documents, validate their content, or to transform other XML formats to CDA documents. XSLT is a pattern based language that makes it very easy to translate one form of XML into another form.

HTML or XHTML – The most common mechanism used to render CDA is to convert it to HTML or XHTML using an XSLT style sheet. The CDA Narrative text model is also very strongly influenced by HTML and its predecessors.

CDA developers will also need to understand a number of other technologies to successfully implement documents. An understanding of these technologies is not necessary to understand this book.

XML Schema – One of the conformance requirements of CDA is that it must validate against the XML schema distributed with the standard.

Schematron – Schematron is a technology that is commonly used to validate the content of a CDA document to ensure that it conforms to the requirements of an implementation guide.

A Note on Key Terms

Standards organizations spend a great deal of time debating the proper terms to use and their definitions. The terms used to describe collections of doctors, nurses, therapists and other personnel employed to provide care to patients are always of particular interest. This book uses the terms in the manner described below:

Clinician – A clinician is a clinically trained and licensed healthcare provider.

Healthcare Provider – A healthcare provider is anyone providing any sort of care to a patient, and may be licensed or unlicensed. Examples of healthcare providers include doctors, nurses, dentists, therapists, and pharmacists.

Provider Organization – A provider organization is a legal entity that engages healthcare providers to provide healthcare goods and services. Examples include a single provider physician or dentist office, a group practice, a hospital, an integrated healthcare delivery network, or a state or local public health office.

The terms are loosely defined on purpose because policies, regulation and law can easily turn one of these entities into another without any regard for the opinions of standards organizations or textbook authors that attempt to rigidly define them.

Editorial Conventions

Quotes from the CDA Standard

Quotes from the CDA standard will be used repeatedly throughout the book. These will appear in this form: [§1.1] to show the origin of the quote.

Quotes from other portions of the standards included in the CDA Normative edition may also appear. These will appear in this form [RIM §1.1]. The abbreviation used will identify the standard in which the quoted text appears. These abbreviations are listed below in

Table 1 Abbreviations for standard references

Abbreviation	Document title
RIM	HL7 Reference Information Model Version
VOC	HL7 Vocabulary Domains
DT	Data Types - Abstract Specification
ITS	XML Implementation Technology Specification - Data Types

Every now and then you will see this symbol on the outer margin. It is used to mark especially *illuminating* text on the standard. The italicized text in that section is a nuance that can help to distinguish one as a CDA expert.

Attributes

The term "attribute" often confuses newcomers to HL7 Version 3 standards. In the context of a class model this term is used to represent members or properties of those classes. For example, a class representing a patient may store the patient's name, gender and birth date. These would be considered class attributes of the patient in the class model.

An XML attribute however, is a specific kind of markup that appears within the XML representation. The class attributes of the HL7 classes can sometimes appear in XML as an element (another kind of markup in XML) or an XML attribute. To avoid confusion, this book with always use the phrase class attribute when talking about the former, and XML attribute when discussing the latter.

Examples

Examples in figures will appear in fixed font. The Italicized text in these examples represents metasyntactic variables that should be replaced by appropriate values. Elision marks (… or :) will appear where material has been removed for clarity.

```
<Element attribute='metaSyntacticVariable' … >
  ⋮
</Element>
```

Fig. 1 Sample example

Sometimes examples of bad practices or invalid XML will be shown, so that you know what to avoid. These examples will be crossed out so that you will not be tempted to use it in applications.

```
<Element attribute='metaSyntacticVariable' … >
  :
</Element>
```

Fig. 2 A bad example

XML element names in the text will be surrounded with pointy brackets and appear in a fixed font like this: `<ClinicalDocument>`.
Attributes names will appear in a fixed font like this: `classCode`

Namespaces

This book contains many examples of XML which demonstrate how a CDA document is represented, or how other XML specifications can be used with CDA. The XML examples contain XML elements that are associated with different XML Schemas (models).

Namespaces are a feature of XML whereby different parts of an XML document can be modeled using different XML schemas. The schemas of each model are associated with a uniform resource identifier or URI (A URI is a generalization of a URL). The namespace itself can be fairly long so they are associated with a namespace prefix.

This book uses the following namespace prefixes in its examples:

Table 2 Namespace prefixes

Prefix	Namespace URI	Description
cda:	urn:hl7-org:v3	CDA Release 2
sdtc:	urn:hl7-org:sdtc	Extensions to CDA maintained by the HL7 Structured Documents Workgroup.
xsi:	http://www.w3.org/2001/XMLSchema-instance	The XML Schema language
xsl:	http://www.w3.org/1999/XSL/Transform	The XML Stylesheet language
ext:	(any)	Arbitrary CDA extensions

HL7 Diagrams

HL7 has a diagramming notation that is explained in more detail in Chap. 12. That diagramming notation relies on both color and shape to convey information. This book is not printed in color, so you will have to rely on the halftones used in it to identify the different HL7 model elements. The figure below shows an example of several shapes in the CDA diagram published by HL7. The text beneath the figure describes how this would be rendered in HL7 diagramming tools.

In HL7 diagrams, the downward pointing arrow labeled **component** is a light pink. The box labeled **Section** that it points to would be a light red or dark pink. The two arrows that point off to the left labeled **author** and **informant** are usually displayed with a cyan and white diagonal pattern, which often appears to be a light cyan. The big arrow labeled **subject** pointing off to the left would be colored cyan (or sky blue). The box it points to labeled **RelatedSubject** would be yellow. The box connected to that one by a straight line labeled SubjectPerson is a bright green. The box on the top left labeled **organization** is usually colored using a diagonal pattern in bright green and white which usually appears as a light green. The box to its right labeled **AssignedEntity** is usually colored using an alternating yellow and white diagonal pattern which appears light yellow.

At the end of each chapter is a chapter summary which highlights the key points of the chapter. Any references to published material will appear following the summary. At the end of each chapter are two sets of questions you can use to test your knowledge of the content in the chapter. The first set include questions that can be answered by reviewing material in the chapter. The second set are research questions which small or medium sized exercises that will help you in your use of the CDA standard. The harder research questions are identified with an * after the question.

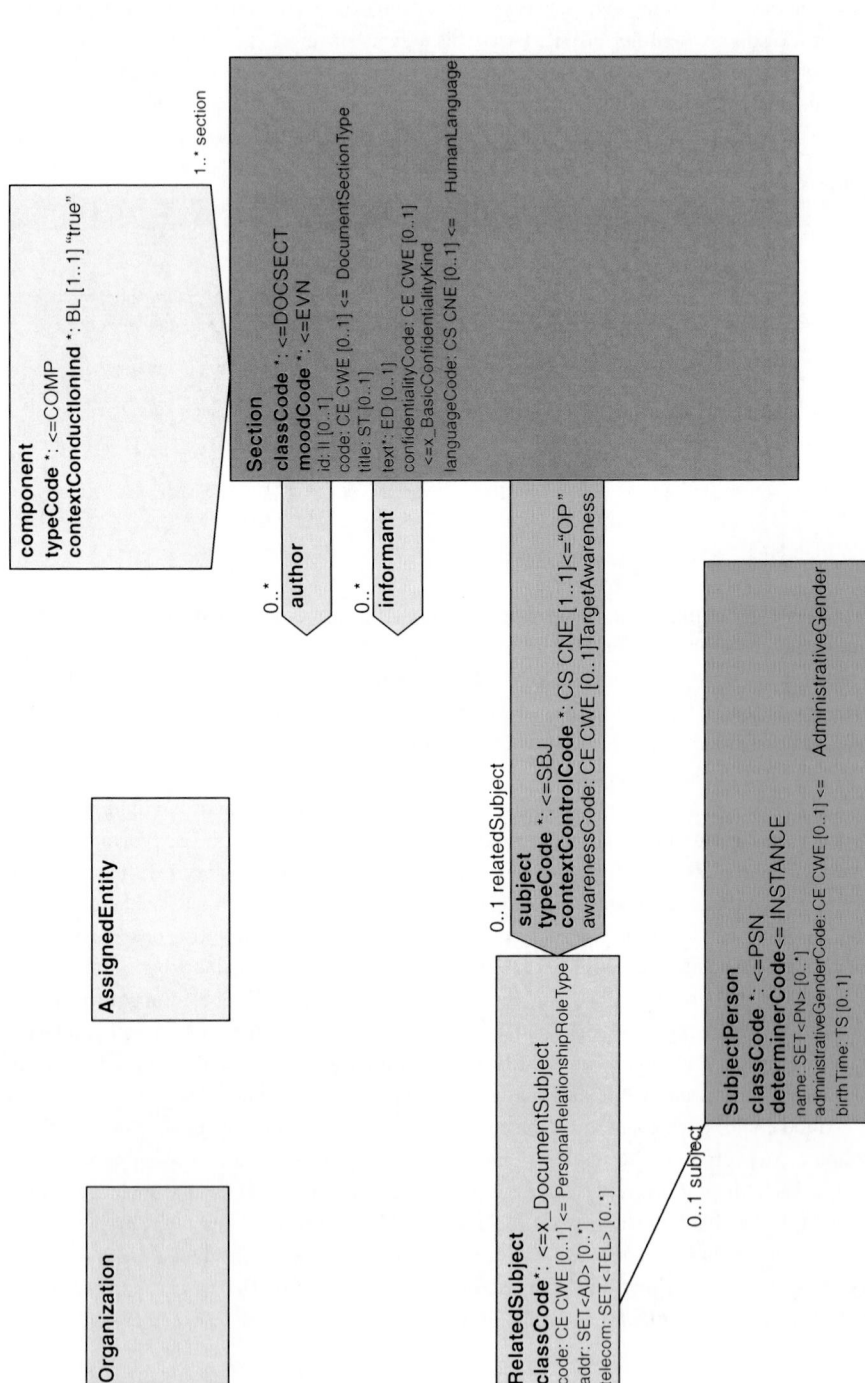

Fig. 3 RIM diagram example

Questions

1. What does HL7 stand for?
2. What does CDA stand for?

Research Questions

1. What is the policy in your region with respect to licensed healthcare providers?
2. How does it differ from policies in nearby regions?*

Acknowledgements

I am extraordinarily blessed by my wife and children, the former who put up with my long disappearances and the latter who gave over their playroom to my writing space in exchange for new bedrooms and other bribes. Among my friends and colleagues, Kate Hamilton of Alschuler Associates, LLC was the chief instigator of this book. Gila Pyke of Cognaissonce deserves a great deal of credit both for cheerleading me on, and reviewing early drafts. Tom DePlonty of InfoExtract is a longstanding friend who demanded to review this book when he heard I was producing it. Both are excellent reviewers who only knew how to spell CDA when they started reading the review chapters. Grahame Grieve deserves a great deal of thanks for a very thorough review of the section on HL7 Data Types.

I am also grateful for the support of HL7 International, especially that of Karen Van Hentenryck who provided assistance obtaining all the necessary permissions to use HL7 content in this book.

Dr. John Halamka was gracious enough to write the introduction for me, and quickly turned it around.

My editor, Grant Weston of Springer-Verlag made a number of suggestions that greatly improved the final text.

I am also grateful that my employer, GE Healthcare has the vision to support healthcare standards.

Finally, while there are too many to recognize individually, I would like to thank all of those volunteers who continue to dedicate their time to the development of standards. I have learned so much from so many of you. Without your efforts, this book would have never been possible.

Keith W. Boone

Contents

Acronyms and Abbreviations

People who work with standards seem to feed on the creation of new acronyms. Since this book is about the Health Level 7 (HL7) Clinical Document Architecture (CDA™), you will rarely see those phrases fully spelled out again. The first introduction of each acronym will be fully spelled out, and the acronym will follow it in parenthesis. A detailed list of all acronyms used in this book and their fully spelled out names and definitions appears below.

ANSI American National Standards Institute ANSI is the US authority with respect to standards.

ASTM ASTM International is an international standards organization formerly known as the American Society for Testing and Materials.

CDA Clinical Document Architecture This book is about the HL7 CDA standard

CMHR Care Management and Health RecordsCMHR is an ANSI/HITSP domain technical committee that writes CDA specifications.

DTD Document Type Definition A DTD is one way to describe content allowed in an XML document.

E31 E31 is the ASTM committee for Healthcare Informatics

HITSP Health Information Technology Standards Panel HITSP was formed in 2005 to select healthcare standards for use by the US healthcare system. ANSI/HITSP completed its federal contracts in early 2010.

HL7 Health Level 7 HL7 is the international standards organization that produced the CDA standard.

HTML Hypertext Markup Language HTML is an application of SGML sometimes used to display CDA documents.

IETF Internet Engineering Task Force

IHE Integrating the Healthcare Enterprise IHE is a profiling organization that produces CDA implementation guides.

ISO International Organization for Standardization ISO is the world's largest standards development organization. It creates international standards across all sectors of commerce.

ITI Information Technology Infrastructure ITI is one of the specialty domains of IHE.

ITS Implementation Technology Specification An ITS is a technical specification that describes how to convert message models based upon the HL7 RIM into the bytes transmitted in an information exchange.

OOD	Object-Oriented Design OOD is a style or method of software design.
PCC	Patient Care Coordination PCC is one of the specialty domains within IHE.
PRA	Patient Record Architecture The PRA was an early name for CDA.
RFC	Request for CommentsThe Internet Engineering Task Force publishes its standards as Requests for Comments. Internet RFCs are available from the web at http://www.ietf.org/rfc.html
RIM	Reference Information Model The RIM is the HL7 representative model for a healthcare system. CDA is based upon the HL7 RIM.
SDTC	Structured Documents Technical Committee SDTC was an earlier name for the SDWG.
SDWG	Structured Documents Workgroup The SDWG is responsible for maintaining the CDA standard.
SGML	Standard Generalized Markup Language SGML was the predecessor to XML
SIG	Special Interest Group A SIG is a type of committee that is devoted to a single topic. HL7 used to convene
TC-215	Technical Committee 215 TC-215 is the ISO Technical Committee for Healthcare Informatics
US TAG	United States Technical Advisory Group to ISO Technical Committee 215 This is a body that represents the US interests to the ISO technical committee on Healthcare Informatics
W3C	World Wide Web Consortium The W3C produces many of the standards used on the web, including XML, HTML and XSLT.
XADES	XML Advanced Digital Electronic SignatureXADES is used to produce a digital signature that can be represented in an XML format.
XHTML	XML Hypertext Markup Language XHTML is a reformulation of HTML following XML markup rules.
XML	Extensible Markup Language XML is a standard markup language that replaced SGML in the late 1990's.
XSD	XML Schema Definition An XSD describes the content allowed in an XML document using the XML Schema language.
XSL	XML Stylesheet Language XSL is a language used to manipulate and render XML documents.
XSLT	XSL for Transformations XSLT is the sublanguage of XSL used to transform information from one XML input format to another output formats using XML, HTML or text.

List of Figures

List of Tables

Introduction

Over the past 7 years, I've facilitated standards harmonization efforts in the United States as the Chair of the ANSI Health Information Technology Standards Panel (HITSP) and the co-chair of the HIT Standards Federal Advisory Committee in the United States.

There a great deal of confusion in the marketplace about standards.

- Are messaging standards obsolete?
- Do document standards contain data or just human readable unstructured text?
- How do the Continuity of Care Record, the Continuity of Care Document and Clinical Document Architecture relate?
- Does the CDA™ standard require a team of PhD's to implement?
- Is a PDF good enough for health information exchange?

Here's my attempt at bringing order to this chaos.

A message such as HL7 version 2 is a transaction used to support workflow between applications within an organization (or between a diagnostic lab and care delivery organization) such as adding a new patient to the registration system, adding a new appointment to a schedule, or posting a new lab result into the patient record. It's transient and not reusable. There are many reasons that a message is still needed to support transactional workflows.

The Continuity of Care Record (CCR) is a fixed number of data elements assembled into a document which describes a transition of care. It's an electronic form of the 3 page Massachusetts Transfer of Care document that is used when a patient is discharged from an acute care facility. It is XML-based and because the number of data elements is limited, it does not require an information model. It does an excellent job of representing one document as XML, but it does not provide an expandable set of data elements or a map of how data elements relate to each other, so it cannot be used to represent all the rich data gathered by payers, providers and patients in all care settings. That's ok, since it was never designed to do so. It's great for transition of care data sharing.

The Clinical Document Architecture (CDA) is an unlimited number of data elements organized by metadata which describes actors, actions, and events in healthcare. It's also XML. The Reference Information Model (RIM) is just a map which relates data elements to each other. The Continuity of Care Document (CCD) is nothing more than the CCR put into CDA XML. In addition to structured data elements, CDA can also represent unstructured text and metadata. CDA is a collection of data elements for healthcare, not a digital version of a paper record.

In many discussions at the HIT Standards Committee, there has been concern about creation of new implementation guides for every possible document in healthcare – discharge summaries, operative notes, histories & physicals etc.

A better way to think about the documents we use in healthcare is as a collection of data elements, in electronic form, capable of many reuses.

CDA is a common container for assembly of structured and unstructured information that does not require creating numerous standards for individual document types.

What has been missing to date is the educational materials to make CDA accessible to everyone. HL7 has been hard at work simplifying CDA. Keith Boone has been hard at work creating this book, which contains the documentation, samples, and guidance needed to successfully implement CDA in real world applications. I'm confident that this book will accelerate adoption of CDA as a means to exchange structured data elements that capture the thought process of the encounter for care coordination but also can be stored as individual data elements for population health, research, and decision support.

Enjoy!

Dr. John Halamka

Organization of This Book

1

The CDA™ standard builds upon the HL7 Version 3 stack of standards. In the lowest layer of that stack are standards on vocabulary and data types. On top of those is the HL7 Reference Information Model.

This book is organized into four major parts. The Introduction describes clinical documents in general, and provides a brief history and overview of the CDA standard. The Data Types part covers each of the data types used by the CDA standard in detail. The Modeling part reviews the HL7 Reference Information Model and its application to the CDA Standard. Finally, the Implementation part covers creation, display, validation of CDA documents and reviews key features of a number of implementation guides that use the CDA standard.

A brief overview of each of the parts and the chapters in those parts should help you to find what you need.

1.1
Part I: Introduction

Chapter 2 Clinical Documentation

This chapter describes the four C's; key properties of clinical documents and from them derives the six key characteristics used in the CDA standard.

Chapter 3 The HL7 Clinical Document Architecture

This chapter provides a brief history of the CDA standard, describes the overall structure of a CDA document, and explains how the standard provides for incremental levels of interoperability.

Chapter 4 Extensible Markup Language

XML is standard for producing structured content similar to what appears in HTML. This chapter provides a brief overview of XML, elements, attributes, the XML declaration, namespaces, XML Schema, parsing technology, and character sets.

K.W. Boone, *The CDA™ Book*,
DOI: 10.1007/978-0-85729-336-7_1, © Springer-Verlag London Limited 2011

Key Terms in the Introduction Part

Clinical Document – A clinical document is typically produced by a clinician and documents clinical observations and services provided to a patient or subject of care.

CDA Document – A CDA document is a clinical document stored in the CDA format. All CDA Documents are clinical documents, but not all clinical documents are CDA documents.

Digital Signature – A digital signature is a collection of data produced by a cryptographic algorithm that can be used as proof that an entity authorized the signature of an electronic document. Note that the US is one of the few countries that allow for both electronic and digital signatures in its laws and regulation. Most other countries with policies on the use of electronic signatures for commerce require the use of digital signatures.

Electronic Signature – In the United States, an electronic signature is defined as "an electronic sound, symbol, or process, attached to or logically associated with a contract or other record and executed or adopted by a person with the intent to sign the record." [1]

Medical Record – A patient's medical record is the collection of documentation used and maintained by a healthcare provider organization to document the care provided to that patient. It is also known as the patient chart.

Semantic Interoperability – The IEEE defines interoperability [2] as "the ability of two or more systems or components to exchange information and to use the information that has been exchanged." Semantic interoperability is focused on the ability to use and understand the information that has been exchanged.

1.2
Part II: Data Types

The most basic components to agree upon in communication are the data types to exchange. The data types used in the CDA standard are defined by the HL7 Version 3 Data Types – Abstract Specification. That specification is described as an abstract specification because it defines the properties, semantics and operations that can be performed on the data types rather than their concrete, computational representations.

The representation of these data types in XML is described in more detail by the XML Implementation Technology Specification included with the CDA Release 2.0 normative edition. This specification makes the implementation of these data types more concrete, and indicates how the information is to be transmitted.

The hierarchy of HL7 Version 3 data types is shown below in Fig. 1.1, along with the subdivisions of this part in which they are covered.

The most important features of commonly encountered data types used in CDA documents are covered in this chapter. More detail can be found in the HL7 Data Types specification. This part is divided into six chapters describing each of the groups of data types shown below.

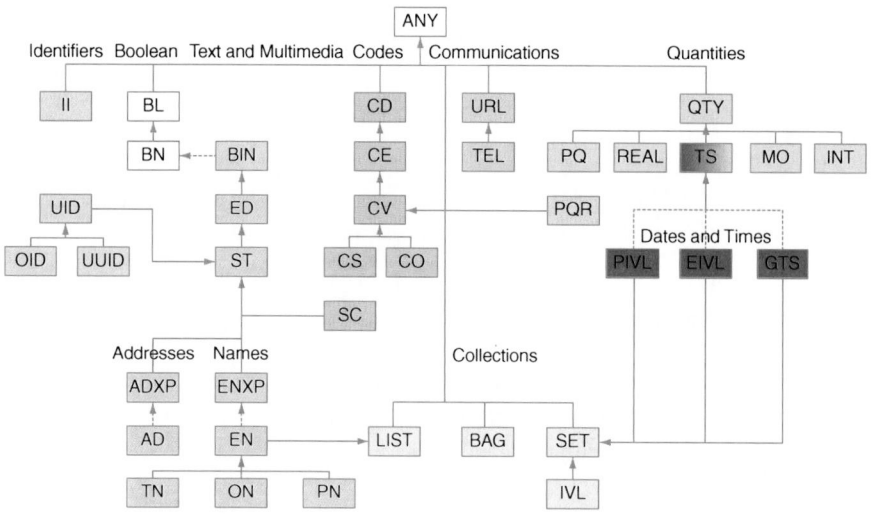

Fig. 1.1 HL7 Version 3 data type hierarchy

Chapter 5   Basic Data Types

This chapter covers the ANY data type and simply valued types including Boolean and numeric quantities. Included in this chapter is a discussion of what HL7 calls flavors of null, which represent the many different reasons why a value is not known.

Chapter 6   Text and Multimedia

This chapter describes how simple strings, text, images and other multimedia content are incorporated into a CDA document using the String (ST) and Encapsulated Data (ED) types. The ED data type supports representation of any kind of multimedia content that has a MIME type associated with it.

Chapter 7   Demographic Data

Demographic data is one of the first things gathered about patients. The eight different data types HL7 uses to support demographic data, including identifiers, names, addresses, telephone numbers and other communication addresses are explained in this chapter.

Chapter 8   Codes and Vocabularies

This chapter introduces the terms used to describe things in HL7 Version 3. It defines key terms such as Concept, Code, Coding System, and Value Set, and explains the difference between pre- and post-coordination. This chapter is an introduces material necessary to understand the following chapter on data types used for codes.

Chapter 9   Codes

Codes represent a concept, or idea. This chapter describe the CD data type and its simpler variants that are used to described codes in the HL7 Version 3 standards.

Chapter 10   Dates and Times

Time is the essence of this chapter. It describes the data types used to capture not just points in time, but intervals over time, and ways to express the timing events that recur periodically. Time is especially important with medications. This chapter shows how to represent the most common medication regimens in the CDA XML.

Chapter 11   Collections

Collections in HL7 are abstract types that can be used to create bags, lists or sets of any data type. This chapter explains what these different types are, and how they work with the HL7 data types representing codes and quantities.

1.3
Part III: CDA Modeling

This part describes HL7 Modeling and how it is applied to the Clinical Document Architecture. It goes on to describe the CDA models for the three different levels of CDA content.

Chapter 12   HL7 Version 3 Modeling

This chapter describes that "language" of HL7 version 3, starting from the six essential RIM backbone classes of HL7 Version 3 which make up clinical statements. It explains the meaning of "mood" as used in HL7 modeling, and how negation works in a clinical statement. Along the way you will learn how HL7 model diagrams are interpreted as UML models, and to interpret the normative representations of the CDA standard.

Chapter 13   Clinical Document Infrastructure

This chapter describes the HL7 model for CDA and discusses features of the XML ITS that are used to generate the CDA XML from this model.

Chapter 14   The CDA Header

Every clinical document has a context that describes the patient, the document author, the related encounter and metadata about the content of the document itself. This chapter describes the RIM classes and XML representations of the CDA header that sets the context for the rest of the CDA document.

Chapter 15   The CDA Body

The CDA body represents the human readable content. In the simplest form of CDA, this is just a file created using traditional documenting tools. But CDA also has a standard format used to encode the narrative. This chapter describes how both of these formats are included in a CDA document, and when the latter form is used, how it can be displayed in a browser using an XSLT transform.

Chapter 16   Clinical Statements in the CDA

The HL7 CDA standard "invented" the notion of a model for clinical statements. This chapter explains what the components of clinical statements are, and how they can be used to represent the machine readable entries in the CDA document.

1.4
Part IV: Implementing CDA

Native support for CDA in applications requires a good bit of restructuring, so the most common way to start generating CDA documents is based on existing application interfaces. These are most commonly implemented using HL7 Version 2 messages. The next step after generating CDA documents is being able to do more than display them. Applications need to be able access the content of CDA documents in meaningful ways.

To simplify application development, CDA can be constrained to support specific use cases. There are a number of techniques that have been used to constrain CDA, and all of these are based on the HL7 Templates DSTU. To support these implementations, application developers need to be able to ensure that the CDA content they receive is valid according to the constraints that have been applied.

A number of organizations, including HL7, IHE, the Continua Health Alliance, the European Smart Open Systems and ANSI/HITSP have created implementation guides using the techniques described previously. The author has been engaged with each of these activities.

Chapter 17   HL7 Version 2 to CDA Release 2

The first place many organizations start when using the CDA standard is creating a CDA document from an existing HL7 Version 2 message. This chapter describes how you can do that for three different types of HL7 Version 2 message most commonly converted into a CDA document.

Chapter 18 Extracting Data from a CDA Document

A document is only useful if it is read. This brief chapter describes a few tools that you can use to "read" the clinical information contained within CDA document. It also explains a technique to access context information associated with a clinical statement using XSLT, which is of the more common information extraction tools.

Chapter 19 Templates

There are more than 100 CDA implementation guides, and more than 500 definitions of CDA components, called templates, that have been defined by these guides. This chapter explains what templates are, the different types, and how they are built. It also explains the meaning of some of the terms used for asserting conformance to a template. Finally, it explains how you can extend CDA to meet requirements that it does not directly support.

Chapter 20 Validating the Content of a CDA Document

This chapter demonstrates some techniques that can be used to ensure that the CDA documents your applications are receiving conform to the rules being defined in CDA templates. It covers four different techniques to validate content, and includes a discussion on validating narrative.

Chapter 21 Implementation Guides on CDA

Work on implementation guides began on CDA Release 2.0 before the ink was even dry on the standard. This chapter explores the history of several important CDA implementation guides. It and describes key features of these guides, and shows how the guides have influenced each other over the years.

Chapter 22 is for you to write.

References

1. Electronic Signatures in Global and National Commerce Act. 15 USC 7001, June 30, 2006. Available on the web at http://frwebgate.access.gpo.gov/cgi-bin/getdoc.cgi?dbname=106_cong_public_laws&docid=f:publ229.106.pdf
2. Institute of Electrical and Electronics Engineers. IEEE Standard Computer Dictionary: A Compilation of IEEE Standard Computer Glossaries. New York, NY: 1990.

Clinical Documentation

2

Clinical documentation is used throughout healthcare to describe care provided to a patient, communicate essential information between healthcare providers and to maintain a patient medical record. What is a clinical document? The simple and easy answer is that a clinical document is anything that you might find in a patient's medical record or anywhere else that documents the care given to that patient.

The definition used by CDA™ for a clinical document is "documentation of clinical observations and services" [§1.1]. This allows just about anything that could appear in a patient's medical record to be a clinical document, but it also allows for other uses. Other documents are also "clinical documents" by this definition, and they need not appear within a patient's medical record. Examples of these include personal health records, public health case reports [1] and quality reports [2] used to track operational activities within a healthcare organization.

Rule #1: My favorite saying among health information management professionals is "If it isn't documented, it didn't happen."

Its corollary is that almost every healthcare activity is documented.

There are other kinds of patients and subjects for which clinical documentation is relevant. Your family pet may have a medical record, and that could contain several different kinds of clinical documents. A friend of mine has a small herd of miniature ponies. That herd could also have a medical record containing several clinical documents. The water in my local pond could also be the subject of clinical observations and services (e.g., number of bacteria of a particular type, and a record of the recent treatment of it). However, CDA Release 2.0 was designed to support clinical documents for human patients, and does not readily support non-human (my cat or my friend's herd) or non-living subjects (the creek in my back yard). CDA Release 3.0 will support clinical documents for non-human patients and non-living subjects. After several years of implementation HL7 has determined that most of the features of CDA Release 2.0 are more than adequate to support these other subjects.

2.1
Properties of Clinical Documents

Clinical documents have two key functions. They **communicate** relevant clinical information between healthcare providers separated by time or distance and support **compliance** with local policy, regulation and law. Key features supporting these functions are **credibility** and **completeness**.

K.W. Boone, *The CDA™ Book*,
DOI: 10.1007/978-0-85729-336-7_2, © Springer-Verlag London Limited 2011

A clinical document must be credible to be effective. This means that it is often produced by a trusted authority and is itself a trusted record of care that was provided.

Clinical documents should also be complete records of care that do not leave out important details. The judgment of what is relevant or important within a clinical document at the time it was written is left to the trusted authorities that produce them. As we learn more, what was important yesterday may no longer be relevant now, but information that seemed irrelevant then might be important today.

These functions and features are intertwined. It would be difficult to provide credible and compliant documentation of care if the documentation were not complete. Similarly an incomplete or non-credible document may result in communication failures that could result in harm to a patient.

2.2
The Six Characteristics of Clinical Documents

 These features and functions lead to the six characteristics of a clinical document defined by the CDA standard. These characteristics are *persistence, stewardship, potential for authentication, context, wholeness and human readability* [§1.1].

Persistence

According to the CDA standard, persistence is a characteristic of a clinical document in that it "… continues to exist in an unaltered state, for a time period defined by local and regulatory requirements." [§1.1]. Healthcare providers and provider organizations are required by local policy, regulation and law to retain documentation of care that has been provided for specific time periods. These time periods can be rather long, for example, patient life plus seven years. One of the reasons for using a standard format for clinical documents is the need to comply with these policies. One need only recall difficulties reading older word processing formats in newer software to understand why a well-documented standard format is needed.

As a result of this characteristic, the CDA standard requires the use of specific versions of the HL7 Reference Information Model, Data Types, Vocabulary and XML Implementation Technology Specification (ITS) be used with the CDA standard. These standards are all subject to updates and maintenance as our understanding of requirements changes over time. Structuring the CDA standard so that specific versions of these standards are used provides a stable foundation. This enables interpretation of the clinical documents conforming to the CDA standard to remain consistent.

The material in this book describes the versions of the foundational standards required by the CDA standard rather than the most current versions of these standards. The foundational standards of the CDA standard are provided in the CDA Release 2.0 Normative Edition, which is available from HL7 International. In large part, the changes which have been made to these foundational standards have been relatively minor in the years since the

CDA Release 2.0 standard was approved. There have been some changes that would have modified the interpretation of a CDA document.

Stewardship

Clinical documents are "maintained by an organization entrusted with its care" [§1.1]. This means that an organization must be able to produce the original of a clinical document, sometimes years after it was created (see Sect. 2.2.1 above). The ability of an organization to produce the original of a document long after it was written aids with compliance and credibility, and ensures that communication can occur long after the patient has left the facility.

The CDA format requires that the name of the steward organization be recorded as of the time the document was created. Over time, organizations may merge with other organizations, may be split off or sold to other organizations. CDA does not require that the history of organizational changes be recorded and maintained after the fact in the document. Instead, it assumes that knowledge of the original steward should be sufficient to locate any subsequent organization that would retain the original copy of the document. The steward of a CDA document is known as its custodian.

The CDA standard does not allow for individual persons to be stewards of documents, only organizations. This would appear to cause difficulty in using the CDA to support clinical documents created by a patient as part of his or her own personal health record. Pragmatically, most of these documents will be stored for the individual by another organization, so this difficulty is readily overcome. Furthermore, nothing prevents an individual person from being represented as an organization in the CDA format. In fact, many single physician practices are sole proprietorships. The legal distinction between the healthcare provider as a person and the organization that they operate is virtually nonexistent. The technical details of the CDA standard are not intended to prevent these providers from creating CDA documents, nor should they prevent patients from creating their own clinical documents using the standard.

Potential for Authentication

The potential for authentication of a clinical document refers to its ability to record or attest to the signature of the legally responsible provider. This legal authentication attests to the completeness and accuracy of the clinical information, and lends credibility to its content.

Clinical documents are often signed by a clinician who takes legal responsibility not only for the content of the document, but also for the acts recorded in that clinical document. The act of legally signing the document does not imply that the signer authored or created the document. For example, an ECG device can create a document containing a patient's ECG readings. The signing clinician may do little more than press a button and enter a password to "sign" the document. There is little authorship involved in this scenario, yet a great deal of responsibility entailed in the signature the clinician attached to the document.

There may be different kinds of "signers" of a clinical document. Some signers are simply attesting that the content of the document is appears as they wrote it. Others are signing the document to assert that not only is it true, correct and complete, but also that that they accept legally responsible for the care described in it. In some jurisdictions, a resident may sign a clinical document to indicate that it documents the care that they provided, but the signature of the patient's attending physician is required to assert legal responsibility for the care.

The CDA standard supports the ability of different types of authenticators to be recorded in the CDA document. It distinguishes between the legal authenticator (the person taking legal responsibility for the document content), and other authenticators.

Legal authentication is recorded in a CDA document a form that supports **electronic signatures** rather than **digital signatures**. An electronic signature is an indelible mark on the bits of the document that assert that the signer did sign the document. A digital signature is a type of electronic signature that uses cryptographic techniques to prove that only the signer could have applied their signature to a document. It is also possible to digitally sign a CDA document, but the standard remains silent on how to accomplish this.

When a paper document is signed, it is very clear that what is being signed is the information that appears on the paper. When a CDA document records the signature of an authenticator, the standard does not make clear that it is the human readable content being authenticated. This is left to local policy for implementation. Other standards and frameworks for electronic and digital signatures indicate that only that which is "seen" should be signed [3].

Organizations using CDA and providing "signed" CDA documents should establish policies on rendering the portions of the document attested to by the signature. The policies on what is attested by a signature may vary between organizations. Healthcare information systems may receive CDA documents from multiple organizations with varying policies with respect to signatures.

Often, organizations will have policies that permit only those documents which have been "legally authenticated" to be accessed by anyone other than the document creator. In these organizations, the act of "signing" the document completes it and makes it available in the patient's electronic medical record. This prevents documents which are still in the process of being written from being used for care before the information in them has been verified by the person legally responsible for the patient's care.

As more health information systems are developed that automatically produce clinical documents, this restriction on release is often relaxed for those automatically produced documents.

Just as organizations do not sign contracts or checks, they also do not sign documents. The authority to sign a document rests with individual people who have been assigned that responsibility by the organization. The CDA standard indicates that the signers of a document are persons, and records the information about the person or persons who signed a document. It also allows for the organizations those persons represent to be communicated. The semantics of the communication make it clear that it is a person who signed the document. The CDA standard supports multiple document signers, but only one person can be recorded as the legal authenticator of a CDA document. Legal authentication applies to the entire human readable portion of the CDA document.

Context

A clinical document tells a story about care being provided to a patient. Like any other story, the clinical document has a particular setting in space and time and a cast of characters that the reader should understand in order to make sense of what has been recorded. These components complete the background associated with the clinical story. This is the context of the clinical document, and it includes:

- The document identifier,
- relevant dates and times associated with the document,
- the type of document,
- the author of the document,
- the legal authenticator,
- the patient (or patients) whose care it describes,
- the clinical encounter and services which it describes,
- any preceding documents it may have replaced or amended,
- the intended recipient of the information at the time the document was written,
- the sources of information contained within the document, and
- the performers of the care described.

This information is stored in the CDA header and provides the default context for all information contained within the body of the document.

The context of the document is also an important feature that enables its retrieval. The clinical documents stored within information retrieval systems are indexed by at least one, and usually more than one of the context components. Health information exchanges are often configured to be able to retrieve clinical documents by this context information. Paper documents are often filed by date of the document and the patient to which they pertain.

Rule #2: If you cannot find a document, it may as well not exist. In which case, see Rule #1.

Wholeness

Like any other story, the story told by the clinical document is more than just the sum of the individual facts and suppositions recorded inside it. Each statement of the story is related to other statements contained in the document. The clinical document may indicate that a certain medication is given to the patient. The statement about the medication is important, but it may not be fully understood without looking at the particular diagnosis, or the set of known drug allergies and intolerances recorded. Thus, a clinical document is legally authenticated as a complete unit of information. The information contained within it is expected to be understood in the context of the whole.

The principle of wholeness does not require the whole content of the document to present to make use of individual statements inside it, but caution is indicated when doing so. Clinical document are often "sliced and diced" to extract and store the clinical statements found inside them. When these statements are stored in separate information systems, they should contain a reference back to clinical document from which they came. This allows users of those clinical statements to access the statements in their original context should any questions arise about them.

Human Readability

Clinical documents are intended to communicate information between healthcare providers. Healthcare providers are humans so clinical documents must be human readable. The principle of human readability means that there must be a way to display the contents of the clinical document in a way that will allow a human to read it. This display can be through a separate application using proprietary formats such as a word processor, or it can be through the narrative format defined in the CDA standard.

This principle means that the CDA standard must support the display of rich multimedia content. While the standard focuses on "reading", that doesn't necessarily mean text. Healthcare providers read graphs and pictures just as often as they read text.

In fact, the multimedia content supported by the standard is much richer that what can be done on paper. It supports audio, video or waveform information as well as narrative text. The key requirement of human readability is that the information supports human consumption.

Several of the developers of the CDA standard started their careers in the realm of technical publishing. The text model they designed in the CDA narrative format supports a model of technical narrative that has been used for decades in electronic publishing. In addition to the traditional hierarchical sections, paragraph, lists and tables, the standard also supports links and footnotes. You can also include links to rich multimedia as separate content, or as embedded and legally authenticated content. The CDA model maps closely to the HTML and XHTML standards from the W3C. Furthermore, it uses the XHTML table model in the CDA XML to support the representation of tables.

One model found in technical publishing that is not found in the CDA narrative model is one of "flows". In publishing, a flow is a continuous stream of text that may be "flowed" into specified portions of the generated output. The CDA standard does not address pagination or rendering issues such as these. These are just another section of text in the CDA document. It is up to the rendering application to determine where the text is placed. Pagination created by the rendering application may include page headers or footers. The CDA standard does not state or directly support document headers or footers, as these are just special kinds of flow objects.

Questions

1. Can a CDA document be used to document care provided to a herd of miniature ponies? A clinical document? Why or why not?
2. What are the four C's of effective clinical documentation?
3. True or False: A clinical document only appears within a patient's medical record.
4. What are the six principal characteristics of a CDA document?
5. What organization is responsible for the development of the CDA standard?

Research Questions

1. How many years must a clinical document be maintained by the organization creating it in your jurisdiction?
2. Who is allowed to legally authenticate (sign) a clinical document in your jurisdiction?
3. What are the legal responsibilities of document signers in your jurisdiction?
4. What is the law in your jurisdiction with respect to electronic or digital signatures?
5. What technologies are required to be used in digital signatures in your jurisdiction?

References

1. HL7 Public Health Case Reporting DSTU, Draft in Development, HL7 International
2. HL7 Implementation Guide for CDA Release 2: Quality Reporting Document Architecture (QRDA), Release 1, April 16, 2009, HL7 International. Available on the web at http://www.hl7.org/documentcenter/ballots/2008sep/downloads/CDAR2_QRDA_R1_DSTU_2009APR.zip
3. XML Signature Syntax and Processing, Second Edition, Section 8.1.2 Only What is "Seen" Should be Signed, June 10, 2008, W3C. Available on the web at http://www.w3.org/TR/xmldsig-core/#sec-Seen

The HL7 Clinical Document Architecture

3

The HL7 Clinical Document Architecture is a standard XML format for clinical documents. This standard is based upon the HL7 Version 3 Reference Information Model (RIM), Data types and Vocabulary standards. The CDA™ standard is also recognized as an ISO and ANSI standard.

The CDA standard is available electronically from HL7 at http://www.hl7.org/implement/standards/. The standard is free to members and available to non-members for a small fee ($50 US at time of publication). The Structured Documents Workgroup (SDWG) of HL7 is responsible for maintenance of the standard, and answering questions about its interpretation. Questions may be addressed to the workgroup through the HL7 e-mail list service. The list service is freely available to anyone. You can sign up for HL7 e-mail lists from at http://www.hl7.org/listservice/. The SDWG holds weekly conference calls which are also open to anyone who wants to participate. You can find the conference call schedule on the HL7 Web site at http://www.hl7.org/concalls.

3.1
History of the Clinical Document Architecture

Figure 3.1 below shows the timeline for the development for the Clinical Document Architecture in HL7.

```
1997 – HL7 SGML SIG begins work on the Patient Record Architecture
1998 – Patient Record Architecture draft
1999 – CDA Release 1.0 Approved by HL7 Membership
2000 – CDA Release 1.0 adopted as an American National Standard
2000 – HL7 XML SIG becomes Structured Documents Technical Committee
2005 – Clinical Document Architecture Release 2 Adopted
2006 – Care Record Summary Implementation Guide
2007 – Continuity of Care Document Implementation Guide
2008 – Recognition of HL7 CDA by the Secretary of HHS
2008 – Submission of CDA to ISO TC-215
2009 – ISO TC-215 Approves CDA as an ISO Standard
2010 – CDA reaffirmed by HL7 and ANSI as an American National Standard
```

Fig. 3.1 CDA timeline

K.W. Boone, *The CDA™ Book*,
DOI: 10.1007/978-0-85729-336-7_3, © Springer-Verlag London Limited 2011

Initial development of the CDA standard started in 1997 through the HL7 SGML Special Interest Group (SIG) of HL7. The SGML SIG later became the SGML/XML SIG while XML was replacing the SGML standard, then it became the XML SIG, the Structured Documents Technical Committee (SDTC), and finally the Structured Documents Workgroup (SDWG), which is how it is known today.

In the early days, CDA was called the Patient Record Architecture (PRA). The first release of the standard was approved by HL7 membership in 1999 and by ANSI in 2000. To achieve ANSI approval, HL7 as an ANSI accredited standards organization, follows its process and informs ANSI upon completion. ANSI then administratively approves the standard as an American National Standard (ANS) after all hurdles are cleared. The first release of CDA was based upon early drafts of the HL7 RIM, Data types and vocabularies. In fact, CDA Release 1.0 is one of the first HL7 Version 3 standards published, preceding the recognition of the HL7 Version 3 RIM, Data Types and Vocabularies standards by 3–4 years.

The second release of the CDA standard was approved by the membership of HL7 in January of 2005 and became an ANSI standard later that year. By that time, the HL7 Version 3 standards upon which CDA is based had been approved by HL7 and ANSI in 2003 and 2004.

Following the adoption of the CDA Release 2.0 standard by HL7, work began on the Care Record Summary Implementation Guide. This was to be a CDA documenting the summary of care provided to a patient. HL7 publication of this document led to a battle between HL7 and ASTM over copyright which was eventually resolved amicably. The resolution of this battle resulted in the co-development of the Continuity of Care Document Implementation Guide by HL7 and ASTM. That implementation guide was approved by HL7 in the following year.

In July of 2008, CDA Release 2.0 was submitted to Technical Committee 215 (TC-215) of the International Organization for Standardization (ISO). It was published as an ISO Standard in November of 2009.

After 5 years as an American National Standard, ANSI required that the CDA standard be reaffirmed, removed or updated. HL7 reaffirmed the CDA standard in January of 2010. CDA Release 3.0 is being developed by the SDWG and is planned for initial balloting in early 2011.

3.2
CDA Is Based on XML

The CDA standard describes the XML elements and attributes that are used to convey clinical information. In CDA Release 1.0, the elements and attributes were specified in the Document Type Definition (DTD) that was provided with the standard. CDA Release 2.0 uses the W3C Schema language to define the elements and attributes of a CDA document. The CDA standard provides the schema in six W3C XML Schema definition (XSD) files.

Unlike other HL7 Version 3 standards, the CDA Schema is a **normative** component [§1.3]. Therefore, XML documents reporting to conform to CDA without any extensions that do not validate against the CDA schema are not valid (see Sect. 20.4 on page 279 for details on how to validate with extensions). *HL7 Version 3 standards normally use the communication models as the normative definition of the standard, and make the XML schemas informative. Both CDA Release 1.0 and Release 2.0 state that a conforming CDA document must be valid against the HL7 supplied schemas. The HL7 CDA schemas therefore are part of the normative definition for the CDA format.*

The CDA standard allows healthcare providers and patients to exchange clinical documents that have been produced from scanned, word processed, dictated, computer entered or electronically generated reports. These reports can be made interoperable at different levels using the CDA standard.

3.3
Structure of a CDA Document

A CDA document is comprised of two parts. The document header sets the context for the clinical document. It contains information such as when the document was written, who wrote it, for what organization, which patient it applies to, and the visit or encounter for which it describes healthcare services. The body of the document contains the human readable narrative text. The term human-readable in this context refers to the ability of a system to render the text in a way that a human can understand its content. It does not mean that the file itself must be in a form that a human could interpret without the aid of some application.

The human-readable text may be stored in a separate file, such as a word processing document or scanned image, or it may appear in a structured format using the CDA XML narrative format. When the document body is supplied in a format other than the CDA narrative format, it is said to be unstructured. While the file formats themselves may be very rigorously structured, the formats are not structured according to the CDA standard.

When the text is stored in the CDA narrative format, it may also include machine-readable information called **entries**. While the entire contents of the CDA are "machine-readable"; the term is used here to refer to the ability of a computer to use these entries to perform functions such as clinical decision support.

The CDA standard has one other restriction on unstructured text. *The file format cannot be XML [§4.3.1.1]* (This is the one question I failed to answer correctly when I reviewed the CDA certification test). The creators of the standard assumed that if you could create XML, you would be able to readily transform that XML to the CDA narrative format. In actual practice, this requirement is often loosened because there is nothing technically that prevents one from putting XML in the non-structured body portion of the document. Some formats cannot be practically translated to the CDA XML format. For example, a rendering of an ECG can be produced using the Scalable Vector Graphics (SVG) format as described in the IHE Request ECG for Display profile.

The SVG format primarily consists of vector graphic rendering commands expressed in XML. CDA does not provide any representation for these commands, and the prohibition this content prevents the image from being included as unstructured content in the body of the CDA document. The transition of word processing formats from binary to XML based formats also makes it difficult to enforce the prohibition. A system supporting CDA documents with word processed inputs becomes non-compliant as soon as the word processor is upgraded to store the information in an XML format. Should the word processor apply a transformation to that XML (e.g., include it in a compressed format that contains a collection of resources, as is the case in the OpenDocument word processing format), the solution becomes compliant again.

3.4
Levels of CDA

CDA Release 1.0 introduced the notion of levels of CDA. Each level introduced a higher degree of semantic interoperability into the exchange of the clinical documents. At Level 1, the CDA provides a collection of metadata used to describe the clinical document, along with the human readable content in application specific or proprietary formats. Level 2 introduces structures to convey the human readable content in a form similar to HTML, and to identify sections of that content using coded terms. Finally, level 3 provides not only human readable semantics, but also machine readable semantic content. These levels are not rigidly defined by the standard. Experts have identified upwards of 12 different shades in between the lowest and highest levels.

Because the CDA standard supports interoperability at multiple levels, it can be implemented incrementally. Scanned document images or word processed documents can readily be exchanged using CDA by simply including them as an unstructured document body inside a CDA Header. Dictated or computer entered text that is available in electronic format can readily be converted directly into the CDA XML narrative format. Finally, electronically generated reports can provide not just human readable, but also machine readable (and semantically interoperable) documents.

Semantic Interoperability is not a switch that you turn on and off. It's a rheostat that you turn up or down.

Summary

- The function of clinical documentation is to communicate between providers and enable compliance with jurisdictional policy.
- Features such as completeness and credibility support the function of clinical documentation.
- The CDA standard identifies persistence, stewardship, potential for authentication, context, wholeness and human readability as the six principal characteristics of clinical documentation.
- The CDA Standard was the first Version 3 standard adopted by HL7.
- A CDA document has a header and a human readable body.
- CDA defines levels of interoperability that support incremental implementation.

Questions

1. What group is responsible for the development of the CDA standard?
2. What are the two parts of a CDA document?
3. What information typically appears in the first part of the CDA document?
4. True or False: All HL7 Version 3 schemas are normative.
5. If you had a question about the CDA standard, what web resource could you use to answer it?
6. What are the characteristics of each of the three levels of CDA implementation?

Extensible Markup Language

4

The CDA™ standard uses Extensible Markup Language (XML) [1] to represent information. XML looks very similar to HTML, but is actually a lower level standard upon which other markup languages are built. XHTML is actually a reformulation of HTML into the XML syntax. HTML allows certain tags to appear with no content. However, XML requires these "empty" tags to be written a slightly different way to indicate that they have no content. HTML also allows attributes without spaced to be unquoted, but XML requires all attributes to be quoted. Figure 4.1 below shows a sample XML document that is used in this section to illustrate the various features of the XML standard.

XML records information using elements, which appear in as text strings surrounded by the pointy brackets < and >.

- The first string inside the pointy bracket is known as the XML element name.
- The first element in the sample document of Fig. 4.1 is the <text> element.
- XML element names usually begin with alphabetic characters, and may contain alphabetic, numeric, underscore, colon, period or hyphen characters [2].

```
<text mediaType='text/x-hl7-text+xml'
   xmlns="urn:hl7-org:v3"
   xmlns:xsi='http://www.w3.org/2001/XMLSchema'
   xsi:type='StrucDoc.Text'
>
   <paragraph ID="para-1">
       This is a paragraph containing text.
       <br></br>
   <br/>
       With two embedded line breaks.
   </paragraph>
</text>
```

Fig. 4.1 A sample XML document

K.W. Boone, *The CDA™ Book*,
DOI: 10.1007/978-0-85729-336-7_4, © Springer-Verlag London Limited 2011

Each element has a beginning and ending point.

- The beginning point of the element is called its start tag.
- Start tags can contain a collection of names with associated values. These are known as XML attributes.
- Attribute names follow the same rules as XML tag names. The attribute name is followed by an equal sign = and then a quoted string, using single ' or " double quote characters.

The quote characters used by XML are characters 34 and 39 of the Unicode character set, also called straight quotes. Some word processors will convert straight quotes to "curly quotes" or "smart quotes" while you are writing. This requires editorial care when writing about XML and XML based standards such as CDA. Developers of CDA implementation guides (and text books) must be very careful to use the right kind of quotation marks in their examples.

The text inside the quoted string is the value of the XML attribute. An XML element can have any number of attributes, but each attribute name can appear only once. In the sample document appearing Fig. 4.1 above, the `<text>` element has four attributes. The name and value of each attribute is shown in the table below.

Table 4.1 Attribute names and values

Attribute name	Attribute value
mediaType	text/x-hl7-text+xml
xmlns	urn:hl7-org:v3
xmlns:xsi	http://www.w3.org/2001/XMLSchema
xsi:type	StrucDoc.Text

Note that the value associated with attribute does not include the surrounding quotes.

Each element start tag must be followed eventually by an end tag. The end tag is like the start tag with a few exceptions. It begins with `</` instead of `<`, and it may not contain any attributes. In between the start tag and end tag is the XML element's content.

The content of an XML element can include:

- other XML elements or
- arbitrary character data, or
- special kinds of XML information such as comments and processing instructions.

An element that has no content can be written using `/>` at the end instead of `>` to indicate that it is empty. The `<br/>` tag in the example above is empty element and is identical in meaning when written `<br><br/>`. XML processors will usually generate the shorter `<br/>` form.

4.1
The XML Declaration

An XML document typically begins with an XML declaration, as shown below in Fig. 4.2. This is sometimes mistakenly called the XML Processing Instruction or XML PI because XML defines a syntax for processing instructions that begins with the <? sequence.

```
<?xml version='1.0' encoding='UTF-8'?>
```

Fig. 4.2 An XML declaration

The XML standard (and the CDA standard) does not require an XML document to begin with an XML declaration. However, it is considered to be a best practice to use one. An XML processor reading a document that starts with an XML declaration can automatically determine the appropriate character encoding to read the rest of the document within a few bytes. It takes no more than 8 bytes to determine enough information about the character encoding to read the complete XML declaration. Having read that, the XML processor can determine the exact encoding from the encoding attribute of the declaration.

version

The version attribute in the XML declaration indicates which version of the XML standard is being used. At the time that CDA Release 2.0 was published, only version 1.0 of the XML standard existed. Since then, the W3C introduced version 1.1. This version is backwards compatible with XML version 1.0. A well-formed XML version 1.0 document can be turned into well-formed XML version 1.1 document by simply changing the version number. In almost all cases the two documents will be parsed identically.

You can represent a CDA document using either XML 1.0 or XML 1.1. The XML ITS is silent on which version of XML to use. However, I would recommend using XML 1.0 unless you are certain you need the features of XML 1.1. Most systems will expect CDA documents to be exchanged using XML version 1.0.

The W3C slightly tweaked the definition of a well-formed document In XML 1.1 to better support the Unicode standard. Many of the reasons to use XML 1.1 are now available in the latest edition of the XML 1.0 standard. The only major features of XML 1.1 which has not been brought back into the most recent edition of the XML 1.0 standard is the support for additional white space characters for line ends supported by some mainframe computer systems.

If you do not know whether you need to use XML 1.1 or not, then you should almost certainly use XML 1.0. The XML standard is now in its fifth edition. Each edition incorporates changes by accumulated errata. One reason cited as a requirement for XML 1.1

had to do with inconsistencies between the XML definition of name start characters and the Unicode definition for ID start characters. This inconsistency was later determined to be an error in the XML specification and was rectified in the fifth edition.

encoding

The encoding attribute of the XML declaration indicates what character encoding is used for the character data in the XML. The character set used internally in the XML standard is Unicode. However, these characters can be represented in an XML document using a number of different character encodings. A character set is an ordered collection of characters, where each character has a unique code. A character encoding describes the rules used to represent the codes used for character in that set. A character set can have more than one encoding. For example, the Unicode character set has three different common encodings: UTF-8, UTF-16, and UTF-32, and a variety of others less commonly used.

According to the XML standard, an XML processor must accept UTF-8 and UTF-16 encodings of Unicode and may accept other character encodings. These may include for example: ASCII, ANSI, ISO Latin-1, EBCDIC or SHIFT-JIS. The XML processor will convert the encodings it recognizes internally to Unicode.

Some Unicode characters may not be able to be directly represented in the text when a document uses an alternate character encoding. For example, there is no character for the Euro symbol € in the ASCII character set. The XML standard requires an XML processor to understand special character sequences known as numeric character references. These sequences are used to represent any character in the Unicode character set.

A numeric character reference:

- begins with an ampersand & and pound (or hash) sign #,
- may contain an x character to indicate use of hexadecimal numbers,
- is followed by a numeric or hexadecimal (if preceded by the x character) representation of the Unicode character, and
- is terminated by a semi-colon ;

Figure 4.3 below shows three different representations of the letter A in an XML document. The last two use numeric character references. The first uses the A character, the second a decimal character reference, and the final one a hexadecimal character reference.

```
A
&#65;
&#x41;
```

Fig. 4.3 Three representations of the letter A in XML

Because the CDA standard is based on XML, it also uses Unicode. Healthcare information systems using the CDA standard must address character encoding issues when extracting and storing information from a CDA document and should document any character encoding limitations.

Many applications do not store Unicode characters natively. System designers should specify how Unicode character data appears that doesn't translate to the encoding system used by the destination information system. Failure to specify this behavior could result in system failures as severe as crashes, and at the very least, can result in unreadable data being stored. Healthcare information systems using CDA to exchange clinical documents should specify what encodings they can accept from other systems and encodings they produce. If you have ever copied text from one application using special characters to another application that does not support them and gotten unexpected and perhaps even confusing results, you should understand the importance of this.

4.2
Namespaces

CDA also makes use of the XML Namespaces [3] standard. The XML Namespace standard describes a mechanism to associate an identifier with the names of XML elements and attributes. This identifier segregates the names of XML elements into different "universes" of names called namespaces. Namespaces are like package names in common programming languages.

The XML Namespace specification supports the use of multiple XML markup language definitions together in one XML document. Each markup language definition can use the same name as is used in another definition, but define it differently. Every element in an XML document is associated with a single namespace. The rules of association defined in the XML namespaces specification make it possible to mix the definitions together.

Namespaces are associated with an XML element through the declaration of a namespace prefix or by declaring the default namespace. The default namespace is assigned by assigning a value to the XML attribute named xmlns. A namespace prefix is declared by adding a special attribute beginning with xmlns: that is followed by a string that obeys the rules of XML element names. The value of this attribute is a URI that uniquely identifies the namespace. A URI is like a URL but can use schemes other than those used by web browsers. Two namespace declarations are equivalent if the URIs that they specify are identical.

Figure 4.4 above shows three namespaces being declared. The first is a default namespace. The next two declarations show that you can have two different namespace prefixes declared using the same namespace.

The default namespace in this example is urn:hl7-org:v3. This namespace is associated with all elements that do not use a namespace prefix. The <text> element above is associated with the default namespace: urn:hl7-org:v3.

```
<text mediaType='text/x-hl7-text+xml'
    xmlns="urn:hl7-org:v3"
    xmlns:xsi='http://www.w3.org/2001/XMLSchema-instance'
    xmlns:xsd='http://www.w3.org/2001/XMLSchema-instance'
    xsi:type='StrucDoc.Text'
  >
```

Fig. 4.4 Namespace declarations

The second namespace declaration associates the namespace URI `http://www.w3.org/2001/XMLSchema-instance` with the `xsi:` prefix. The third namespace associates that same namespace with the prefix `xsd:`.

The final attribute in this example (`xsi:type`) is associated with the namespace that has the URI of `http://www.w3.org/2001/XMLSchema-instance`. It would not be legal to include an attribute named `xsd:type` in this element because the two prefixes `xsi:` and `xsd:` refer to the same URI. This would result in an element that has two identically named attributes. To associate an attribute with a namespace you must use a namespace prefix, as attributes do not use the default namespace.

The URIs associated with namespaces are sometimes associated with web accessible resources that define the specific XML markup language used. These resources often provide that definition in an XML markup language known as the XML Schema Language.

All CDA instances must define at least one namespace (`urn:hl7-org:v3`) because that is the namespace associated with the CDA schema. All elements defined by the CDA standard must appear in that namespace. I recommend using this as the default namespace because it simplifies implementations. Most CDA instances will also define a namespace for `http://www.w3.org/2001/XMLSchema-instance`. This namespace defines a `type` attribute that allows the data type to be further specified when necessary (see Abstract Types on page 36 for more details).

4.3
XML Schema Language

The XML Schema Language [4] is a language used to define XML markup languages. It is itself an XML markup language, which can lead to interesting circular definitions that amuse computer geeks. CDA Release 2.0 is a markup language for clinical documents that is defined using this standard. The CDA standard defines a number of defaults associated with documents communicated using it and makes it a requirement of receivers to assume these defaults if the information is not transmitted [§1.3.1 Recipient Responsibilities]. *The easiest way to ensure that your application assumes these default values is to parse the document with schema validation enabled. This will automatically insert the default values for you into the parsed document.*

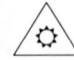

The URI associated with CDA Release 2.0 is `urn:hl7-org:v3`. A conforming CDA Release 2.0 document must therefore include a namespace declaration. Figures 4.5 and 4.6 below show two different ways to include the declaration of the necessary namespace.

Figure 4.5 uses a default namespace declaration. This is the preferred method of many implementers because it eliminates extra characters in the resulting document. I personally

```
<?xml version='1.0' encoding='UTF-8'?>
<ClinicalDocument   xmlns="urn:hl7-org:v3"
    xmlns:xsi='http://www.w3.org/2001/XMLSchema-instance'>
...
</ClinicalDocument>
```

Fig. 4.5 CDA document with a default namespace declaration

```
<?xml version='1.0' encoding='UTF-8'?>
<cda:ClinicalDocument xmlns:cda="urn:hl7-org:v3"
    xmlns:xsi='http://www.w3.org/2001/XMLSchema-instance'>
...
</cda:ClinicalDocument>
```

Fig. 4.6 CDA Document with a prefixed namespace declaration

prefer this form when creating CDA documents in an implementation. It simply requires less typing.

Figure 4.6 uses a prefixed namespace declaration. Other implementers prefer this method because it clearly identifies CDA elements. CDA implementation guide authors often use this form because CDA is used with other XML standards, and it makes it clear which standard you are using (I often use this form in implementation guides for the reason stated). The name used for the prefix does not matter to the XML processor, but conventionally either cda: or hl7: is used as the prefix.

Implementations should never try to force the use of any particular method for declaring the namespace. While it might be nice if everybody did it the same way, it does not matter to the XML processor. In many cases it is nearly impossible to control what prefixes are used in a CDA document generated by an application.

Use of xsi:type

All of the namespace examples you have seen thus far declare the http://www.w3.org/2001/XMLSchema-instance namespace. The XML Schema [5] standard defines this namespace. This namespace defines the meaning of four attributes that can be used in XML documents: *The last two of these are NOT permitted to be used in CDA documents according to [§ITS 1.4].*

Attribute	Purpose
type	Allows for explicit specification of the type of an XML element.
nil	Declares that an element should be considered valid even though it has no content.
~~schemaLocation~~	Declares the location of the schema associated with a particular namespace.
~~noNamespaceSchemaLocation~~	Declares the location of a schema that is not associated with a particular namespace.

The namespace is usually associated with the xsi: prefix. The xsi:type attribute is often needed by CDA implementers. One of the most important XML elements in the CDA standard requires that you further specify the data type associated with the XML element before you use it. The <value> element used in observations is defined in the CDA standard to be of the ANY data type. This means that you must promote it to one of the concrete CDA data types to report the value of any observation. Other XML elements in the CDA standards have a default data type associated with them, but can be promoted to a more specific data type. Type promotion requires the use of the xsi:type attribute.

```
<value xsi:type='PQ' value='300' unit='mg'
   xmlns='urn:hl7-org:v3'/>
<cda:value xsi:type='cda:PQ' value='300' unit='mg'
   xmlns:cda='urn:hl7-org:v3'/>
```

Fig. 4.7 Use of xsi:type with namespace prefixes

In order to promote a CDA element to a specific data type, you include the name of the data type as the value of the xsi:type attribute, as shown in the examples in Fig. 4.7.

These examples illustrate a very important fact about type names. The names of the data types use the same prefixes as the names of CDA elements in the XML document. Applications using the type of an XML element have to be carefully written to ensure that they look for the correct type name depending upon the namespace declarations in effect in the document. Recall that the same namespace can be declared with two different prefixes. Thus, if both the hl7: and cda: prefixes are associated with urn:hl7-org:v3 as is the default namespace, then the PQ data type could be named PQ, cda:PQ or hl7:PQ in the XML representation. This is shown in the example in Fig. 4.8. below.

```
<cda:observation xmlns:cda='urn:hl7-org:v3'
xmlns:hl7='urn:hl7-org:v3'>
   ...
   <cda:value xsi:type='cda:PQ' value='300' unit='mg' />
   <hl7:value xsi:type='hl7:PQ' value='300' unit='mg' />
</cda:observation>
```

Fig. 4.8 Use of xsi:type with multiple namespace prefixes

Do Not Use the schemaLocation Attribute

While the XML Schema Language allows a schema location to be associated with an XML document by including a schemaLocation attribute associated with the http://www.w3.org/2001/XMLSchema-instance namespace, this is explicitly PROHIBITED by [ITS§1.4], and thus by the CDA standard.

Systems validating a CDA document are expected to provide their own schemas to use during validation. This rule is sometimes broken by CDA implementers. Applications receiving CDA documents should at the very least REMOVE the schemaLocation attribute from the document before processing it, if not rejecting documents containing them completely. Downloading schema resources from arbitrary URLs or file locations for validation can at the very least slow down your system, and could crash it or even worse, cause a security breach. I have seen a number of different systems crash at testing events upon seeing an otherwise valid CDA document containing a `schemaLocation` attribute pointing to a file that does not exist.

4.4
Parsing the CDA XML

Almost every programming environment supports an XML parser these days, from the most common to the most obscure. Finding a parser for your CDA implementation project will not be difficult. What might be difficult is choosing between them. An old joke I heard in computer sales circles was the customer pitch: "You can have high quality, great features and low cost – which two do you want?" The same is pretty much true for any high-end solution. However, once that solution becomes commoditized, you can get all three. That is what has happened with XML parsing technology. I divide features up into two main categories: speed and extensibility in the analysis below.

Parser Quality

The quality of the parser can have a large impact on a CDA implementation project. Fortunately, there are a large number of very well tested high-quality XML parser implementations in just about every programming language. Because XML parsing is a commodity technology, a product that has been around for a while and has a recent release is a good indicator of implementation quality.

Speed

Speed is a big concern when you consider that a medium sized suburban hospital can generate three million or more clinical documents a year. However, the development of service oriented architectures, virtualization technology and increased hardware capacities make speed less of a concern when scalable implementation architectures are used. It is only when chokepoints are introduced where all CDA documents have to flow through systems with limited resources that speed needs to be the primary concern.

There are three principal methods of processing XML, event based processing using the Simple API for XML (SAX), object oriented processing using the Document Object Model (DOM), and query based methods which use XPath, XQuery or similar query capabilities against an XML data store.

Event driven parsing reads the XML and generates events through which processing actions can be triggered. Event driven parsing applications can be automatically generated by software and can generate high throughput implementations. However, even driven processing models are difficult to work with when multiple parts of the clinical document need to be accessed at the same time (e.g., when collecting and comparing problem lists).

Object oriented processing models often use event driven parsing to build a complete in memory representation of the XML document. In memory representations are very effective when different parts of the document need to be accessed simultaneously for processing, but are often much slower than event driven processing.

Efficient serialization of the data structures found in an XML document can often reduce performance issues by eliminating reparsing of the document as it is processed. Query based processing models rely on efficient serialization of XML on storage devices. The query based models store the document in a data store that is optimized for XML-based information. Repeated processing of the document no longer requires parsing once it has been stored in the system. Efficient queries can then be used to access different parts of the document. This also allows access to different parts of the document at the same time. Query based processing methods are effective when the same document needs to be processed repeatedly by multiple systems (e.g., when performing analysis through multiple processing stages).

The W3C is recently completed work on a standard for Efficient XML representation. This representation will allow for efficient storage and communication of XML documents. Documents stored in this format can be processed much faster than in the original XML in text format. Eventual deployment of XML processors which support this format will dramatically improve XML based implementations in the future.

Extensibility

One very common form of XML processing that is used with CDA is transformation of the CDA XML to other formats. This is most often accomplished using a processor supporting the XML Stylesheet Language for Transformation (XSLT). XSLT processors use a pattern/action model of transformation. The XSLT standard defines how patterns are matched in the input (using the XPath standard), and describes the desired end result to be generated when those patterns are matched. This is a declarative programming model rather than a procedural model. In a procedural programming model, you describe the operations that generate the end result, rather than describing the end result directly.

Getting used to the declarative programming model can be difficult at first. This difficulty is usually overcome with practice as users discover the nuances and common idioms of the language. In fact, the declarative programming model can accomplish all the same tasks that a procedural one can. However, it is sometimes just plain easier, more efficient or comprehensible to write procedural code. It is important then to use an XSLT processor that can be integrated with a procedural language. Almost all common XSLT processors can do so, but this can also restrict your choice of programming language. If you chose an XSLT processor from a particular supplier, you will often be limited to the favorite programming environments and languages of that supplier.

EXSLT is a vendor neutral set of XSLT extension specifications. These extensions often eliminate the need for writing platform specific code in your transformations. EXSLT is supported by many common XSLT parsers, and you can readily find implementations for the common XML parsers that do not support it natively. You can find the EXSLT documentation and downloads on the web at http://www.exslt.org/.

Another useful feature of an XML parser is the ability to query the parsed document model using a standard query language like XPath or XQuery. This capability is available in more mainstream programming environments. If you are developing in one of those "odd-duck" environments you may need to look carefully to find an XPath and/or XQuery capability that works for you.

Cost

Cost of an XML processor is probably the least of your concerns. Due to the abundance of freely available XML parsing tools, you will be able to find most of what you need for free. However, as a colleague of mine often notes, less than 25% of the cost of software is in the acquisition of it. Three quarters or more is in dealing with maintenance, deployment and integration of that software into your environment. These other costs can be reduced by paying attention to quality, speed and extensibility.

Summary

- CDA relies upon W3C XML, XML Namespaces and XML Schema standards.
- CDA documents are stored using Unicode characters.
- Namespace declarations are required inside CDA documents.
- Certain features of the XML standards must be used with care, and others are prohibited.
- High quality, low cost XML Parsers are readily available for just about all programming languages and environments.

Questions

1. What does an XML declaration tell the XML processor?
2. What are the differences between HTML and XML?
3. What would a namespace declaration for a CDA document look like?
4. How can you ensure that your XML processor applies the defaults specified in the CDA standard?
5. Why does the namespace associated with the URI `http://www.w3.org/2001/XMLSchema-instance` need to be declared in a CDA document?
6. How would a PQ data type be named in an `xsi:type` attribute if the namespace declaration for `urn:hl7-org:v3` used the `cda:` prefix?
7. Why must the `xsi:schemaLocation` attribute never be used in a production system?

Research Questions

1. XML developers commonly develop conventions for use of single quotes, double quotes, prefixes associated with namespace declarations, character encodings and use of XML declarations. What would your authoring conventions look like and why?
2. What character encodings does the XML processor you use support?
3. What versions of XML does your XML processor support?
4. How do you enable schema validation in your XML processor?
5. *What namespace declaration should be used for CDA Release 1.0?
6. *What edition of XML version 1.0 does your XML processor support?

References

1. Extensible Markup Language 1.0 (Fifth Edition), November 26, 2008, W3C. Available from the web at http://www.w3.org/TR/xml
2. Ibid, Section 2.3 Common Syntactic Constructs
3. Namespaces in XML 1.0 (Second Edition), August 16, 2006, W3C. Available from the web at http://www.w3.org/TR/xml-names/
4. XML Schema Part 0: Primer Second Edition, October 28, 2004, W3C. Available from the web at http://www.w3.org/TR/xmlschema-0/
5. XML Schema Part 1: Structures Second Edition, October 28, 2004, W3C. Available from the web at http://www.w3.org/TR/xmlschema-1

Basic Data Types

5

5.1
ANY

All of the HL7 Version 3 data types derive their properties from the ANY data type. Common features of all of the data types are implemented here. For example, almost all HL7 data types can indicate that the value is unknown. This property is implemented in the CDA™ schema through the ANY data type.

Having a singly rooted hierarchy for data types also allows for elements in the CDA XML to be declared that support any arbitrarily selected HL7 data type. Observations about a patient can take on any of the different data types. The data type is not known until the type of the observation is specified, so the <value> element of the CDA <observation> is specified to be of this type.

nullFlavor

HL7 Version 3 has more to say than many other environments that deal with unknown values. Most environments have only one way to say unknown, but the HL7 CDA standards supports 11 different ways to say this. You not only indicate that something is null, you can also say why. *This particular feature of a null value is called its flavor of null.*

Most applications do little with the various flavors of null in current implementations. These are most useful in reasoning applications that can change their logic depending upon why the information is not present.

There are 11 flavors of null appearing in HL7 Version 3, although 12 appear in the edition provided with CDA Release 2. These appear in Table 5.1 on the following page along with an explanation of their meaning. The complete specification for nullFlavor appears in [DT§2.1.1]. The four in bold often appear in CDA specifications and CDA documents. The last one flavor of null is never used CDA documents, and was subsequently removed from the HL7 RIM. All of the others appear infrequently.

K.W. Boone, *The CDA™ Book*,
DOI: 10.1007/978-0-85729-336-7_5, © Springer-Verlag London Limited 2011

Abstract Types and xsi:type

The HL7 Data Types specification defines several abstract types including the ANY and QTY data types. These data types support common properties found in the data types that are derived from them, but are not meant to exist in the world without more concrete definition. An abstract definition is therefore "incomplete" and cannot stand on its own.

Abstract types can be used to define a schema for XML instances, but cannot be used within an XML instance. The purpose that they serve in the schema is to stand for their more derived counterparts. Because these are defined to be abstract in the XML schema, an XML parser will not know the exact data type that is represented in an XML document without a further "hint". This hint is provided to the XML parser in the form of a type declaration using the `xsi:type` attribute on the XML element. The two examples in the figure below show the use of this XML attribute to indicate use an Integer for the `<value>` element.

The name of the data type is given as the value of the `xsi:type` attribute. Data type names use the same namespace prefix as the CDA document. If you use `urn:hl7-org:v3` as the default namespace, as in the first example, then the name of the Integer data type is `INT`. However if the namespace uses another prefix value as in the second case, the name of the Integer data type is preceded by that namespace prefix (`cda:INT` in this example).

```
<value xsi:type='INT' value='1'/>
<cda:value xsi:type='cda:INT' value='1'/>
```

Fig. 5.1 Using `xsi:type`

Other Uses of xsi:type

The xsi:type attribute is also used in a few other cases where several choices exist for an element. For example, the `<effectiveTime>` element underneath the `<substanceAdministration>` is defined to be of type SXCM_TS. This data type supports a wide variety of different ways to specify dates, ranges, intervals and repeating time periods. The simplest is to just express the time as a timestamp, which needs no further action. However, to express more complex times, you need to use one of the data types derived from SXCM_TS (for example, IVL_TS). In this case, you would use `xsi:type` to specify the more derived type.

Table 5.1 Flavors of NULL

Null flavor	Explanation
NI	If you see this, it basically means that the value isn't there, and that's all the more you will know.
OTH	Use this value when you KNOW the code doesn't exist (e.g., a code for the novel H1N1 virus strain of swine flu in SNOMED CT before November of 2009), or when it isn't present in the allowed set of values you are constrained to provide. This is typically used with coded data types.
NINF PINF	Negative and Positive infinity only applies to numeric data types such as INT, PQ or REAL. These can be used with interval data types (IVL_*) to indicate an unbounded lower or upper bound. They do not apply codes, strings, Booleans or other data types.
UNK	This means "I don't know".
ASKU	This means "I don't know but I did try to find out"
NAV	This means "Not available" which can be translated into "I don't know right now, please ask again later".
NASK	This means "I don't know and I did NOT try to find out"
TRC	This means an inconsequential amount greater than zero, and should be used with PQ or REAL, since it does indicate a quantity.
MSK	This often indicates that sensitive information is being hidden. It is rarely used in CDA implementations.
NA	This means that a value is not applicable.
NP	This value indicates that the value is not present in a message, and should be replaced with the default value. This flavor of NULL is NEVER used in CDA and has been removed from current implementations of the RIM.

Contents of this table are drawn from the HL7 Vocabulary Standard with permission. Column 1 comes directly from the standard. Column 2 is the author's interpretation.

The `<value>` element found in `<observation>` elements in the CDA schema is defined to be of the ANY data type. To specify that the `<value>` of an `<observation>` is unknown, the example in Fig. 5.2 would seem to be sufficient; **but this representation is not legal**.

```
<value nullFlavor='UNK'/>
```

Fig. 5.2 Incorrect use of nullFlavor in `<value>` elements

The example in Fig. 5.3 shows the correct way to represent an unknown value in a CDA document. To correctly represent the unknown value, you must specify the data type of the `<value>` element.

```
<value nullFlavor='UNK' xsi:type='PQ'/>
```

Fig. 5.3 Correct use of nullFlavor in `<value>` element

Why is the data type required when the value is unknown? The simple answer is that this is a mistake that was made during the definition of the original ANY data type created in the HL7 Abstract Data Types specification. According to [DT§1.11]: This is an abstract type, meaning that no value can be just a data value without belonging to any concrete type. The consequence of defining ANY to be abstract was carried through in [ITS§2.1], which explicitly states: *ANY is an abstract datatype and may not be used directly; hence, ANY* has no XML representation.

The problem introduced by making ANY abstract is that you are forced to select a data type, even though you may not know which one would be appropriate (This problem has been corrected in the HL7 Data Types Release 2.0 standard). However, CDA documents must always indicate the data type of the `<value>` element by supplying an `xsi:type` attribute. So, when the data type of a `<value>` element is unknown, how should it be represented? The answer may appear in several places. Senders of CDA documents should use other available sources (e.g., implementation guides) to determine the appropriate data type to use. When the implementation guide does not offer an answer, use the most generic concrete data type you can when supplied with multiple choices. If all else fails, make a logical choice. In all cases ensure that the behavior is well documented. As a receiver, you should not rely on the expressed data type of an element when it records an unknown value.

5.2
Booleans

Usually there is only one Boolean data type in programming language. However, HL7 has more to say than most because of the use of flavors of null. A typical Boolean value can have one of two non-exceptional values. HL7 Version 3 uses the values "true" and "false" to represent the two usual cases.

Most Boolean class attributes in the HL7 CDA Class diagram will be represented as XML attributes in a CDA document as shown in the example below.

```
<entryRelationship inversionInd='true' ...' >
```

Fig. 5.4 Boolean data types used in XML attributes

However, Booleans are also often used to deal with simple "yes/no" or "true/false" answers to questions, and so may appear in a `<value>` element in an observation. In these cases, the value of the Boolean variable appears in the `value` attribute of that element.

```
<value xsi:type='BL' value='false'>
```

Fig. 5.5 Boolean data types as an XML element

HL7 has two different kinds of Boolean data types, which are described in further detail below.

BL Boolean

The vanilla Boolean data type has two non-exceptional values: `true` and `false`. It can also represent any of the various flavors of null. The BL data type is used in the `<separatableInd>` in `<entryRelationship>` and `<reference>` elements, in the `<preferenceInd>` element of the `<languageCommunication>` element, and in the `<independentInd>` element of the `<supply>` element.

BN BooleanNonNull

The `BooleanNonNull` data type is a little more traditional, in that it can only represent `true` or `false` values. If you don't know, don't try to say it with a `BooleanNonNull`, because you simply cannot. This data type is not meant to be used by itself, but only as part of larger data types.

5.3
Quantities

Quantities are most often used in CDA documents to report numerical measurements in clinical observations. Quantities are numeric, and can also have units of measure (common) or currency denominations (rare) associated with them. Most quantities found in a CDA document will appear in `<value>` elements in observations (`<observation>`), reference ranges (`<observationRange>`) or the preconditions (`<precondition>`) associated with clinical statements.

Quantities also appear in a few other places in the CDA schema to report an ordinal sequence number (the numerical position) of an item in a list. These quantities will always use the Integer data type.

QTY Quantity

All numeric data types derive from the Quantity (QTY) data type. This data type is abstract, just like the ANY data type. Abstract types cannot be directly used within a CDA document.

The HL7 data type specification uses this data type to represent common properties of all numeric data types. These properties require that comparison operations (equal, less than, greater than), and addition and subtraction operations be defined on any concrete data type derived from quantity.

In order to define addition and subtraction operations, one must be able to specify the data type used to represent differences between any two instances of the data type. Common numeric types such as INT and REAL use the same data type (INT and REAL respectively) to represent differences. However, the Timestamp (TS) data type uses the physical quantity (PQ) data type to represent the difference between two time stamps as some real quantity of time units (e.g., seconds, minutes, etc.).

INT Integer

The integer data type represents a positive or negative integer or zero. Negative integers are preceded with a minus sign. Positive integers may be preceded by a + sign, but need not be. The Integer (INT) data type is used sparingly in the CDA schema. It appears in the <sequenceNumber> element of the <entryRelationship> and <component> elements, and in the <versionNumber> element of <ClinicalDocument>, <externalDocument> and <parentDocument> elements.

It also is used in the <value> element of <observation> elements to record observations that are simple integers without any attached units. When used in the <value> element of an <observation>, the xsi:type attribute must be specified. Figure 5.6 below shows use of the INT data type in the <value> element, along with the proper specification that this data type is being used in the xsi:type attribute. Note that xsi:type requires the use of the same namespace as is used for elements in the CDA instance.

```
<value xsi:type='INT' value='1'/>
<cda:value xsi:type='cda:INT' value='1'/>
```

Fig. 5.6 INT data type in <value>

REAL Real

The real data type follows from INT, save that it contains positive or negative real numbers or zero, rather than just integers. Real numbers appear in the value attribute as either

decimal numbers or double precision floating point numbers in the XML. These representations are described in more detail in the definition of decimal and double data types in
sections 3.2.3 and 3.2.5 of XML Schema Part 2: Datatypes Second Edition.

PQ Physical Quantity

A physical quantity has two main components, a value representing the magnitude of the
measure, and the units in which the item is measured. The PQ data type is very much like
a vector in mathematics and has many of the same properties of vectors. Most physical
quantities simply are vectors, but a few are not. Some physical quantities represent measures on a scale that does not have vector properties.

The PQ data type is most often used in the `<value>` element of the `<observation>`,
`<observationRange>` or `<precondition>` elements. Recall that the `<value>`
element is declared in the CDA schema to be of the ANY data type in these classes. The
PQ data type must be explicitly assigned to this element using the `xsi:type` attribute as
shown in the figure below.

```
<value xsi:type='PQ' value='200' unit='mg'/>
```

Fig. 5.7 Use of PQ data type in a `<value>` element

The PQ data type also appears in the `<quantity>` element of the `<supply>`
element. It is also used with Intervals (described in the next section) in the
`<doseQuantity>`, `<rateQuantity>` and `<maxDoseQuanity>` elements of the
`<substanceAdministration>` element.

value

The value attribute represents the magnitude of the measurement. It must appear as a decimal number or a double precision floating point number.

unit

The unit attribute contains a code from the Unified Code for Units of Measure (UCUM)
describing the units (the dimension) in which the physical quantity is measured. The HL7
Data Types specification requires the use of UCUM [1] for the representation of units. This
attribute must be present when the quantity being measured is not a simple count of things
(e.g., caplets, cells or other objects without an associated unit of measure)

The UCUM code system is maintained by The Regenstrief Institute, and is freely available
for anyone to use. UCUM supports the representation of units of measure with less ambiguity
than existing combinations of ISO and ANSI units currently used in HL7 Version 2 standards.

Some common units of measure appearing in UCUM are shown in the table below.

Table 5.2 Example UCUM units

UCUM unit	Meaning	UCUM unit	Meaning
m	Meter	kg	kilogram
[in_us]	US Inch	[lb_us]	US pound
L	liter	g/l	grams per liter
mL/(8.h)	Milliliters per 8 hours	m/s²	meter per second squared

UCUM is an interesting code system because it defines the rules by which codes are created using a formal grammar, rather than enumerating all possible values. This makes the UCUM code system infinite in size. A simplified grammar using Augmented Backus-Naur Form [2] appears in the figure on the next page. In this grammar, a `prefix` is any symbol found in table 1 or 23 of the UCUM standard (about 25 symbols), and an `atom` is any symbol found in tables 2 through 22 of the standard (almost 300 in all).

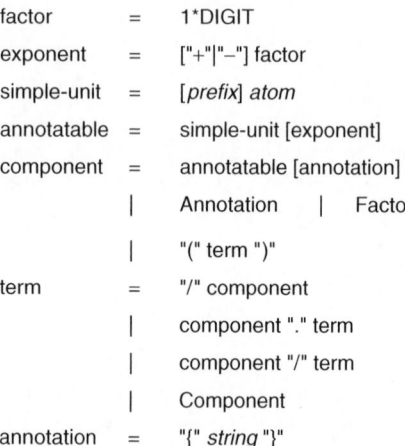

factor	=	1*DIGIT
exponent	=	["+"|"−"] factor
simple-unit	=	[*prefix*] *atom*
annotatable	=	simple-unit [exponent]
component	=	annotatable [annotation]
	|	Annotation | Factor
	|	"(" term ")"
term	=	"/" component
	|	component "." term
	|	component "/" term
	|	Component
annotation	=	"{" *string* "}"

Fig. 5.8 ABNF grammar for UCUM

If you are building a parser for UCUM, you should be aware that two "special" atoms in UCUM begin with a digit sequence: "10^" and "10*". These atoms represent the dimensionless constant 10. These atoms allow for compact representations of 10 to any integer power. When these sequences are found they must be treated as the atomic unit, rather than a digit sequence followed by a * or ^ sign.

UCUM defines codes for six units: meter, gram, second, radian, Kelvin, Coulomb and candela. These are used to measure length, weight, time, angle, temperature, charge and luminous intensity respectively in the standard. All other units are defined (eventually) in terms of these base units. Units may be composed of other units by using multiplication or division operations (using. or /). Units may also be raised to an integer power, or multiplied or divided by an integer.

Some UCUM units can be preceded by a metric prefix (e.g., producing kg for kilogram from k for kilo and g for gram). UCUM defines a table of common prefixes in section 4.1 of the standard. This table includes all third powers of 10 between 10^{-24} and 10^{24} and every power of 10 from 0.001 to 1000. Symbols for typical ANSI units of measure (e.g., inch, ounce and pound) do not allow metric prefixes; there is no "kilo-inch". However, there is a Kibit. UCUM defines four prefixes: Ki, Mi, Gi and Ti (2^{10}, 2^{20}, 2^{30} and 2^{40} respectively) to represent common powers of 2 related to computer technology measures (bit, By, and Bd for bit, byte and baud respectively).

The UCUM standard provides eight pieces of information in tables in the standard for each atomic unit. These are:

- The name of the unit,
- a description of what it measures,
- a print or display name,
- a case sensitive code,
- a case insensitive code,
- a flag indicating whether or not the unit takes metric prefixes,
- a constant scalar value
- a unit expression or conversion function

The last two columns in the tables describe how a unit is derived ultimately from one of the base units. To translate the physical quantity from one unit expression to another, you replace the unit in the original expression with the unit it is derived from, and multiply the magnitude by the scalar value.

The representation in the figure below can be translated to centimeters as using Table 8 found in section 34 of the UCUM standard.

```
<value xsi:type='PQ' value='6' unit='[ft_i]'/>
```

That table defines a [ft_i] as being 12 [in_i], and defines [in_i] as being 2.54 cm. To perform the translation, of 6 [ft_i] to meters, first multiply 6 by 12, and replace [ft_i] with ([in_i]), giving 72 ([in_i]). Next, multiply 72 by 2.54, and replace [in_i] with (cm), giving 182.88 ((cm)).

This expressive power of UCUM means that there can be several codes representing functionally equivalent concepts. A couple of examples of this are shown in the table below.

Table 5.3 UCUM equivalents

Functional equivalents	UCUM code	Concept represented
Newton	N	Newton
	kg.m/s2	kilogram-meter per second^2
	kg.m.s-2	kilogram-meter second^{-2}
Kilometer	km	Kilometer
	10*3.m	10^3 meters
	1000.m	1000 meters

The UCUM standard provides the information necessary to recognize these different codes as being functionally equivalent.

Neither UCUM nor the HL7 Physical Quantity data type defines a canonical representation for physical quantity expressions. They simply note that a canonical representation can be generated from any appropriate set using all the dimensions of measure described previously. Two unit expressions are *commensurate* if they measure the same thing, e.g., length, velocity, weight, force, etc. When two unit expressions are commensurate, they can be compared to each other. There are several commercial and open sources that can handle UCUM and can convert and compare between commensurate units.

IVL_* Numeric Intervals

The HL7 Data Types specification describes an interval as continuous range in an ordered base type (e.g., Integer, Real, Physical Quantity or Time Stamp). All ordered base types in the HL7 Data Types specification conveniently are derived from the Quantity (QTY) data type. A fully specified interval has a lower and upper boundary (either of which may be infinite). A fully specified interval that has non-infinite boundaries also has a center point (defined as the arithmetic mean of the lower and upper bound), and a width (defined as the difference between the upper and lower bound. Given any two of these values, the other two can be determined when the interval is not infinite. This would allow for ten representations in the XML.

The XML Implementation technology specification only allows for the following eight representations of an interval to be used:

- <low>
- <width>
- <high>
- <low> <width>
- <width> <high>
- <low> <high>
- <center>
- <center> <width>

Most CDA implementation guides restrict the representation of intervals to an even smaller number of forms. The most common restrictions allow for only: <low> by itself, <high> by itself or both <low> and <high> elements.

There are times when only one aspect of the interval is known (e.g., the start or end, or the width). An incompletely specified interval is legal to use in a CDA document. For example, when a medication is specified, often the dosing instructions are written as "take three times a day for 10 days." Neither the starting nor ending times for taking the medication are present in this instruction, so you can only record the width of the interval. The HL7 Claims Attachment Implementation guides use this feature to record the number of days that a medication should be taken.

Another example where <width> is important is where the start date and duration of a procedure is known, but the start and stop times for the procedure are not known to sufficient precision to compute a useful width. For example, a procedure occurring on April 26th, 2010, taking 45 min might best be represented using a <low> and <width> form.

<low>, <high>

These elements define one of the boundaries of the interval. If the interval is of type IVL_T, then this element is derived from type T, where T could be any of INT, REAL, PQ or TS. The actual type in the schema is IVXB_T, which adds the inclusive XML attribute to the base type. The value XML attribute in this element contains the boundary of the interval.

```
<value xsi:type='IVL_INT'>
   <low value='1' />
   <high value='3'/>
</value>
<doseQuanity xsi:type='IVL_PQ'>
   <low value='7.5' unit='ml'/>
   <high value='15' unit='ml'/>
</doseQuantity>
<time xsi:type='IVL_TS'>
   <low value='20100701'/>
   <high value='20100818'/>
</time>
```

Fig. 5.9 <low> and <high> examples

inclusive

The inclusive XML attribute appears on the <low> or <high> element where needed to specify whether this boundary point is included (the default) or excluded from the interval. It is rarely used in CDA documents.

<center>

The <center> element describes the arithmetic mean of the interval boundaries. When the interval is of type IVL_T, the <center> element is of type T, where T could be any of INT, REAL, PQ or TS. This implies that the center may not be able to be represented when using IVL_INT, because the arithmetic mean may not be an integer (Actual use of IVL_INT is rare in the real world, so this is not a big problem). Also note that if the width of the interval is infinite (either of its endpoints are at positive or negative infinity), it has no center.

<width>

The <width> element describes the width of the interval using the difference type associated with the type of the interval. If the interval is of type IVL_*T*, then <width> is of type DIFF.*T*. For Intervals over the types INT, REAL or PQ, the difference type will be the same as the base type. When the interval is over time (i.e., IVL_TS), the <width> element will be of type PQ with a time based unit. The units of that physical quantity will be some measure of time (e.g., hours, minutes or seconds).

```
<value xsi:type='IVL_INT'>
   <center value='2' />
   <width value='2'/>
</value>
<doseQuanity xsi:type='IVL_PQ'>
   <center value='11.25' unit='ml'/>
   <high value='7.5' unit='ml'/>
</doseQuantity>
<time xsi:type='IVL_TS'>
   <center value='20100725'/>
   <width value='50' unit='d'/>
</time>
```

Fig. 5.10 <center> and <width> examples

Summary

- The ANY data type is the root of all HL7 data types.
- Almost all HL7 data types support the expression of unknown values through the nullFlavor XML attribute.
- Booleans come in two forms, the BL data type which supports unknown values, and the BooleanNonNull or BN data type which does not.
- The quantity data type is the root of all numeric data types.
- The REAL data type is represented the same way real numbers are represented in the W3C Schema specification.
- Physical Quantities act like vectors, with the magnitude given in the value XML attribute and the dimension given in the unit XML attribute.

Questions

1. How do you represent an unknown value in a CDA document?
2. What else must you specify with the `<value>` element when it is unknown?
3. Why are there two different Boolean data types in the CDA specification?
4. Where are the two different ways a real number can be represented in a REAL data type defined?
5. Is the following element legal in a CDA document? **`<value xsi:type='QTY' value='10'/>`**
6. What unit does the code [fur_us]/2.w represent?
7. Represent the interval shown below in all legal forms. What form cannot be used and why?

```
<value xsi:type='IVL_INT'>
    <low value='1'/><high value='4'/>
</value>
```

Research Questions

1. Find or implement a parser for UCUM and describe how it works.
2. Describe two different sets of units that could be used to define a canonical form for units.
3. Which units do not represent real dimensions in a vector space?
4. What sort of clinical statement could require an open interval in its representation in a CDA document?

References

1. Unified Codes for Units of Measure, 2009, Regenstrief Institute, Inc. Available on the web at http://aurora.regenstrief.org/~ucum/ucum.html
2. RFC 5234 Augmented BNF for Syntax Specifications: ABNF, January 2008, Internet Engineering Task Force. Available on the web at http://www.ietf.org/rfc/rfc5234.txt

Text and Multimedia

6

6.1
BIN Binary

The binary data type is a collection of raw bits. HL7 treats this conceptually as a list of BooleanNonNull values. An empty stream of binary data is considered to be an exceptional (null) value. The binary data type is an abstract one, which means that this data type is cannot be used inside a CDA™ document. To send binary data see Encapsulated Data below.

6.2
ED Encapsulated Data

Encapsulated data is the way that HL7 transmits data in formats not defined by HL7. This data type can include images, video, audio, waveforms, genetic sequences, multimedia, et cetera. Encapsulated data can appear in a CDA in one of two ways. The data may be referenced (by a URL), or the data may be directly incorporated into the CDA document.

The most frequent use of the ED data type is in `<text>` elements found in either `<section>` elements of the CDA document or in various clinical statement elements (see Clinical Statements on page 188). Encapsulated data is also placed in `<value>` elements of the `<observationMedia>` element of a CDA document to store multimedia data associated with the clinical document. It may also appear in the `<value>` element of an `<observation>` to store multimedia data such as a genomic sequence stored in a standard (but non-HL7) format. It also appears in `<text>` elements of clinical statements and in the `<originalText>` elements of coded data.

representation

CDA data is transmitted in XML, but multimedia content is often in binary and needs to be translated into a text format before being embedded in the XML content of a CDA document. The `representation` attribute of the ED data type allows the CDA document to indicate whether the content is text, or a base-64 encoding of the data.

K.W. Boone, *The CDA™ Book*,
DOI: 10.1007/978-0-85729-336-7_6, © Springer-Verlag London Limited 2011

```
<observationMedia representation='TXT'>
taaccctaat tactcttact caaccatggc aaactctcct cctcctcatc
attctcctct
</observationMedia>
<observationMedia representation='B64'>
     VGhpcyBpcyBCYXNlLTY0IGVuY29kZWQgdGV4dC4NCg==
</observationMedia>
```

Fig. 6.1 Example ED data type representations

The default representation is text, and so need not be supplied when the data can be directly included in the XML of the document. Data that is base-64 encoded must use the encoding defined in RFC 2045.

TXT – This value indicates that the data is in a text format. This is the default format.

B64 – This value indicates that the data is based 64 encoded according to RFC 2045.

Use of XML in Encapsulated Data

According to the definition of the ED data type in [ITS§2.5]: … ED can contain the data as XML markup. In these cases the mediaType is expected to describe some form of XML markup, and the content must be well-formed XML contained in a single element in the ED content.

BASE 64 Encoding

Base-64 encoding uses one text character to store six bits of raw data. Base-64 encoding is like hexadecimal encoding, but using 64 different characters for the digits 0-63 (the letters A-Z, a-z, numbers 0-9, plus +, slash / and equals =). If you were counting, you realized that was 65 characters. The equals sign is used as a delimiter to mark the end of a transmission and may appear more than once depending on how many bits have been transmitted.

The base-64 following depicts the encoding of the ASCII string: This is Base-64 encoded text.

VGhpcyBpcyBCYXNlLTY0IGVuY29kZWQgdGV4dC4NCg==

Base 64 encoded data is usually transmitted with line breaks after every 76th character to make the encoded data more palatable (and not just for humans, some transmission networks still have problems with lines longer than 80 characters). Characters not in the base 64 character set are ignored in base 64 encoded data so these extra line breaks do not result in decoding errors.

This makes it clear that an ED is capable of including XML content directly within the CDA document in an element using this data type as shown in the example below.

```
<value xsi:type='ED'>
  <foreign:other>
      ...
  </foreign:other>
</value>
```

Fig. 6.2 Using the ED data type to store non-CDA XML

However, CDA documents that are written to take advantage of the capability to include XML defined outside of the HL7 CDA schema will not be valid according to the schemas that come with the CDA standard. This does not mean that this feature is not allowed, it is simply not supported in the schema. It does imply that fewer uses of it will be encountered in real-world implementations that use the CDA standard.

To take advantage of this capability and use a schema you must alter the schemas provided by HL7. If you want to include XML elements from other schemas the definition for the ED data type must be altered in the schema. The definition for this data type is found in the `datatypes-base.xsd` file that comes with the CDA standard. The schema definition for it is shown in Fig. 6.3 with the necessary addition shown in bold type (This example does not include the schema annotation for the sake of brevity). This alteration has been proposed for the next release of the HL7 normative edition. This will not affect CDA Release 2.0, but would provide better support for what the ITS allows in future HL7 Version 3 standards, including CDA Release 3.0.

These changes do not fully restrict the legal values appearing inside the ED data type to those allowed by the standard. This is because of limitations of the XML Schema language. The ED data type uses what is called a mixed content model. The mixed content model is required because the ED data type contains other elements that describe the encapsulated data, including the `<reference>` and the `<thumbnail>` elements.

```
<xs:complexType name="ED" mixed="true">
  <xs:complexContent>
    <xs:extension base="BIN">
      <xs:sequence>
        <xs:element name="reference" type="TEL"
           minOccurs="0" maxOccurs="1"/>
        <xs:element name="thumbnail" minOccurs="0"
           maxOccurs="1" type="thumbnail"/>
        <xs:any namespace="##other" minOccurs="0"
           maxOccurs="1" processContents="skip"/>
      </xs:sequence>
          ...
    </xs:extension>
  </xs:complexContent>
</xs:complexType>
```

Fig. 6.3 Modifying the ED data type to store non-CDA XML

`<xs:any`	This element allows for unspecified elements to appear within an instance.
`namespace="##other"`	Allows the element to appear in any namespace except `urn:hl7-org:v3`.
`minOccurs="0"`	Indicates that the element need not appear (it is optional).
`maxOccurs="1"`	Indicates that no more than one may appear.
`processContents="skip"`	Indicates that the foreign element will not be validated. You may also use the value `strict` but then you will need to `include` the foreign schema within `cda.xsd`.
`/>`	

Fig. 6.4 Explanation for schema change

mediaType

The `mediaType` is stored as an XML attribute on the encapsulated data element. This type must be a MIME media type. The XML ITS standard makes recommendations in [ITS§2.5.3] about media types that are required, recommended and deprecated. In practice, any MIME media type is permissible, and the HL7 deprecated types are often ignored. The default `mediaType` is text/plain.

The `<text>` *element of the CDA* `<section>` *uses the encapsulated data type and fixes the XML* mediaType *attribute to* `text/x-hl7-text+xml`. *That means that the narrative text of the clinical document is stored as multimedia text. There are some thoughts in the Structured Documents Working Group that the HL7 narrative format should be replaced by a standard format such as XHTML in CDA Release 3.0.*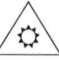

charset

The `charset` XML attribute appears in elements of the ED data type to indicate the character set and character encoding used for text based content. Legal values for this attribute are defined by the Internet Assigned Numbers Authority (IANA) and can be found in http://www.iana.org/assignments/character-sets.

The `charset` attribute is only relevant when used with references to external content or with base-64 encoded content. This attribute does not apply to inline data that has not been base-64 encoded. That is because the XML document already specifies the character encoding of the XML content, and the character encoding cannot be altered inside the document.

language

The language XML attribute appears in elements of the ED data type to hint at the language used for text based content. This is transmitted to enable applications to better present or display the text. It could for example, trigger the loading of appropriate language libraries to enable text to speech translation of the embedded text. This attribute can safely be ignored.

compression

The compression XML attribute appears in elements of the ED data type to indicate the form of compression that has been used on the data. This XML attribute is only used if the compression being performed on the data is not already part of the specification for the content. For example, GIF and JPEG images are already stored in compressed form, and so would not be compressed again.

Base 64 encoding of data increases transmission size of encapsulated data by a factor 4:3 in the most commonly used encodings, and can increase the size by 11:4 using UTF-16 or even as much as 11:2 for UCS-32.

Reducing the size of the encapsulated data by using data compression can recover some of that lost bandwidth. Several compression algorithms are available, including deflate (see RFC 1951), gzip (see RFC 1952), zlib (see RFC 1950) and the old Unix compress algorithm (deprecated due to use of patented algorithms).

Compression of data occurs before data is base 64 encoded (and decompression after it is decoded). Data that is already in a compressed format (newer word processing and image formats) will not benefit from compression, but uncompressed formats such as TIFF or BMP or text-based formats such as XML or RTF almost certainly will.

Table 6.1 on the following page shows the codes that must be used for each compression algorithm.

Table 6.1 Compression algorithm codes

Code	Compression algorithm	Specification
DF	Deflate	RFC 1951
GZ	GZip	RFC 1952
ZL	ZLib	RFC 1950
Z	Compress	Deprecated

Implementations must support the Deflate algorithm and may support the other three, although Compress is deprecated by HL7. This is due to patents and efficiency. Other algorithms are faster, publicly available and implemented in common programming environments.

Compression

Every 77 characters transmitted in base 64 encoded format will result in about 57 bytes of raw data. When the XML is encoded using an 8-bit character set, or in UTF-8, the data will consume about 1.3 times the storage as the original raw file. However, when using a 16-bit character set (e.g., using the UTF-16 encoding), it will take about 2.7 times the storage.

Compressing the encapsulated data can reduce the amount of storage that is consumed. The TIFF, RTF and XML based multimedia formats benefit greatly from compression. Compression does not usually impact more recent multimedia formats since they are already compressed.

<reference> (see TEL on page 75)

Another way to transmit binary data is to provide a reference to a location where it can be obtained (e.g., a URL to an image). When the encapsulated data is provided through a reference the element containing the encapsulated data will contain a `<reference>` element. This element uses the TEL data type (see page 75 below) to record the URL containing the data in the `value` attribute.

Applications must be careful when processing elements that contain `<reference>` *elements. The* `<reference>` *element must never be preceded or followed by additional whitespace. This whitespace can be interpreted as the inline data representation of the content.*

When using just the `<reference>` element, it should be written as shown in the example below:

```
<text><reference value='#fragment-id'/></text>
```

Fig. 6.5 Correct use of `<reference>`

The `value` attribute contains the URI for the referenced text and may be a relative or absolute URI. The example above also illustrates a common pattern used in CDA specifications. The `<reference>` contains a URI that points to the text that should be used. A URL is a special type of URI that is familiar to users of the Internet.

A URL usually points to a resource that you can access on the web. Figure 6.6 below shows an example of a URL.

```
http://sample.org/path/resource#fragment
```

Fig. 6.6 A sample URL

This example is made up of the components described in Table 6.2 below. An absolute URL like the example above includes all components except the fragment identifier (which is optional). Relative URLs omit components from the left hand side. When components are omitted, the processor of the URL assumes they have the same values as the resource currently being accessed.

Table 6.2 URL components

Component	Example	Description
Scheme	`http://`	The URL Scheme used to determine how to access the resource (e.g., the world wide web, file transfer, a local file, et cetera.)
Hostname	`sample.org/`	The hostname where the resource is stored.
Path	`path/`	The path to the resource
Resource Name	`resource`	The resource name
Fragment Identifier	`#fragment`	An identifier of a component inside the resource

In the example in Fig. 6.5, only the fragment identifier is provided. In this case, the CDA document is the resource being accessed. The fragment identifier indicates which part of the document should be located. Different MIME types can specify the meaning of the fragment identifier. MIME types based on XML use fragment identifiers to locate the XML element containing the specified fragment identifier in an XML ID attribute. The CDA Narrative text schema found in NarrativeBlock.xsd includes an ID attribute on all text components found in sections. The CDA schema itself also adds this attribute to `<observationMedia>` *and* `<section>` *elements.*

The use of `<reference>` elements containing fragment identifiers is heavily used in implementation guides of CDA that use machine readable entries. There are at least two different reasons for this approach.

1. References point back to the original text rather than repeat it
2. The reference acts as a direct link between the machine readable entries to the narrative content to which it applies.

Pointing to text avoids duplication of it in the document and ensures that the same text is used everywhere. The question of how to interpret a clinical document where the narrative said one thing but the machine readable portion said something else never arises.

Linking the text to the machine readable entry supports better identification and understanding of content. Without these links a consumer of a CDA document only knows that the entries appear in some portion of the narrative text appearing in the section, but will not know which part. The linking of machine readable entries to narrative text can also be used by rendering tools to provide additional capabilities, such as pop-up windows that provide details found in the machine readable portion of the text.

The `<reference>` elements should not have any additional white space added before or after them (this is because they use Mixed Content Model, described in the sidebar on page 63). The next example shows an incorrect use of the <reference> element illustrating this. In this example, the <reference> element is preceded and followed by extra whitespace (newlines and spaces).

```
<text>
    <reference value='#fragment-id'/>
</text>
```

Fig. 6.7 Incorrect use of <reference>

According to [DT§2.4.5]: An encapsulated data value may have both inline data and a reference. The reference must point to the same data as provided inline.

As a result, any text (whitespace or otherwise) appearing within an element of the ED data type it is expected to be part of the inline text representation. The use of more than one contiguous piece of text in the element to represent the data is prohibited by [ITS§2.5] where it states: An instance of *ED* may only contain at most one text node (A piece of contiguous text is called a text node in the XML standard.).

References are prohibited in some places in the CDA specification. For example, the <text> element of a <section> cannot be provided using a <reference> element. In other cases the encapsulated data can only be provided by reference. When a <text> element appears inside of the <parentDocument> element, it must contain only a <reference> element. The CDA document is not permitted to directly contain the text of the document that it is related to.

According to [DT§2.5.7]: An encapsulated data value may have both inline data and a reference. The reference must point to the same data as provided inline.

The content of the URI pointing to this element must exactly match the data provided inline in the CDA document. Unless otherwise restricted, the <reference> element can appear with the inline text data.

Why would you duplicate text contained within an online resource? A perfect use case for this is demonstrated above in this book. I have duplicated snippets of text found in the various HL7 standards, as well as provided a reference to where you can find them. The same case could also be applied to clinical documents. The author of the document may want to include the referenced text to make it easier for people to access the information, and reference it so that the reader can verify for themselves what was actually said.

If you use this capability, you must be wary of inserting extra whitespace into the XML representation. Additional whitespace appearing between the <reference> element and the inline data will be taken as part of the inline data. I recommend use of either the <reference> element or the inline data, but not both due to this issue.

The examples below show two different representations of an ED data type used to contain the text string This is some sample text. The first example is correct. The second and third examples are incorrect.

```
<value xsi:type='ED'><reference
value='http://sample.org/sampletext'>This is some
sample text</value>
```

Fig. 6.8 Correct use of `<reference>` and inline data

```
<value xsi:type='ED'>
        <reference value='http://sample.org/sampletext'>
        This is some sample text
</value>
```

Fig. 6.9 Incorrect use of `<reference>` and inline data

```
<value xsi:type='ED'><reference
value='http://sample.org/sampletext'>
This is some sample text</value>
```

Fig. 6.10 Another incorrect use of `<reference>` and inline data

The example of Fig. 6.9 is incorrect because the `<value>` element contains two pieces of text and the `<reference>` element as well additional whitespace not in the original text. The first piece of text is the whitespace appearing between the `<value>` element and the `<reference>` element. While this text is only whitespace, there is no way to tell that this text is not relevant. The second piece of text contains additional whitespace characters (XML treats newlines as whitespace) both following the reference element and before the `</value>` end tag.

The example of Fig. 6.10 is wrong because even though it has eliminated the whitespace between the `<value>` start tag and the `<reference>` element and before the `</value>` end tag there is still the extra newline appearing after the `<reference>` element.

integrityCheck

The `integrityCheck` XML attribute appearing in the element representing the ED data type is a secure hash value over the data contained within it. This value is base-64 encoded before it is placed in the XML attribute. This XML attribute supports verification that content appearing in a reference has not been altered since it was used in the document.

integrityCheckAlgorithm

The `integrityCheckAlgorithm` XML attribute indicates which algorithm was used to produce the `integrityCheck` XML attribute value. This XML attribute may contain the value SHA-1 or SHA-256 depending upon which algorithm was used. If not specified, the hash algorithm used is assumed to be SHA-1.

thumbnail

Thumbnails are smaller forms of images or content which are used to represent the full data. A thumbnail can be used very much like an icon. These are represented in a `<thumbnail>` element that is itself of the ED data type. This element is restricted in that it cannot contain another `<thumbnail>`.

6.3
ST String

The string data type is perhaps the easiest to understand. It encodes simple text data.

This data type is represented in HL7 Data Types as a constraint on the ED data type. The XML attributes for `representation` and `mediaType` are fixed to the values TXT and text/plain respectively.

There are no references, integrity checks or thumbnails for these simple text strings. The `language` XML attribute is used just as described above for the ED data type. There is no need to record the character set information since the text is incorporated into the XML document using the character set specified in the XML declaration of the CDA document.

```
<value xsi:type='ST'>A String</value>
```

Fig. 6.11 ST data type example

Note that neither of the following examples are correct for sending an empty string.

```
<value xsi:type='ST'></value>
<value xsi:type='ST'/>
```

Fig. 6.12 The wrong way to send an empty string

Instead you must send a flavor of null, as shown in the example below.

```
<value xsi:type='ST' nullFlavor='UNK'/>
```

Fig. 6.13 The right way to send an empty string

The same rules also apply when sending an empty ED data type.

Summary

- The Encapsulated Data (ED) data type supports the inclusion of multimedia content in CDA.
- The stream of bits found in the Encapsulated Data type is represented as text, XML or as base-64 encoded content in the text.
- The `<reference>` element requires special care when being used to represent a link to the actual text.
- The CDA `<text>` element found in `<section>` elements use the ED data type with a fixed media type and XML representation.
- Strings (ST) are constrained from the ED data type.

Questions

1. What is the `mediaType` for the example provided below?

```
<observationMedia representation='TXT'>
taaccctaat tactcttact caaccatggc aaactctcct
cctcctcatc attctcctct</observationMedia>
```

2. What character set is used to represent information contained within elements using the String (ST) data type?
3. V2hhdCBpcyB0aGUgdGV4dCBvZiB0aGlzIHF1ZXN0aW9uPw0K
4. Is the following a legal rendition of the ED data type?

```
<value xsi:type='ED'
>Some text<
reference value='http://127.0.0.1/text'/
></value>
```

Research Questions

1. What other schema definition languages might be used to further restrict the content of the Encapsulated Data (ED) type to the set of legal values permitted by the XML ITS?
2. Compute how much space is "wasted" using the Base 64 representation for Encapsulated Data in the XML. How much of this space could be regained by compressing the data for different media types?

Demographic Data

7

CDA™ provides eight different data types to record what is commonly thought of as demographic data. These are address parts and addresses; name parts; organization, personal and other names; identifiers, and telecommunications endpoints.

7.1
ADXP Address Part

Postal addresses can be parsed into a collection of different parts. Each of these parts identifies a geographic or political boundary at some level of detail. The CDA standard supports the identification of more than 25 different parts of a postal address, including parts such as a house or building number, direction indicator on a street, post box number, and apartment number. These more detailed address parts are infrequently used inside CDA documents. CDA implementations should be prepared to specify how addresses must be represented in documents that are exchanged, or to handle them in all of their complexity.

Without looking at the CDA standard, how many different parts of a postal address can you come up with?

partType

Each address part is assigned a code called the address part type. This code is stored in the `partType` attribute in the CDA schema. Implementations usually do not typically use the `partType` attribute. The value of this attribute is fixed for each of the different elements used to markup parts of an address. The CDA schema automatically supplies the appropriate value for this attribute when these elements appear.

Health information systems traditionally divide an address up into one or more street address lines; a city; state, province, territory or similar division; postal code and may also support country and county, parish or similar division. In the United States, 49 states have counties and the state of Louisiana uses the term parish. The term parish is also used in other countries such as United Kingdom and Ireland.

K.W. Boone, *The CDA™ Book*,
DOI: 10.1007/978-0-85729-336-7_7, © Springer-Verlag London Limited 2011

<deliveryAddressLine>

The <deliveryAddressLine> is intended to record parts of an address like post office box numbers, rural routes and general delivery addresses. These are used for the delivery of correspondence, but do not correspond to the physical location of the recipient. It is rarely used for this purpose as most CDA implementations use the <streetAddressLine> element for this purpose. This is because most information systems do not distinguish between a delivery and a street addresses.

<streetAddressLine>

The <streetAddressLine> element is intended to record a physical street address. This address may be used to deliver correspondence or to physically locate the destination. As previously noted, the CDA standard allows this element to be repeated as many times as needed. While most healthcare information systems support more than one street address line, few support more than three, and some healthcare standards such as X12N support only two lines for an address.

<city>

The <city> element records the city, town or other municipality associated with the address. In the new release of HL7 data types expected to be used with CDA Release 3.0, the city can be bound to a list of legal values.

<state>

The <state> element records the state, province, territory or similar geopolitical boundary. In HL7 Data Types Release 2 (expected to be used with CDA Release 3.0) the state can be bound to a list of legal values.

<postalCode>

The <postalCode> element records codes used and defined by the delivery agent to identify the delivery or street address. In the US these are known as ZIP codes, and this US-centric view is reflected in the code used to identify this address part.

<country>

The <country> element records the country. HL7 Data Types Release 2 will allow the country can be bound to a list of legal values. ISO 3166 Part 1 defines one such list of country codes. Implementations should be prepared to deal with the fact that geopolitical boundaries change (For example, in 1993, the country of Czechoslovakia was subdivided into the Czech Republic and Slovakia). ISO 3166 Part 3 contains historical country names which should also be supported in a binding of this element to a code list.

<county>

The <county> element records the country, parish or similar subdivision. It is often used in addresses associated with healthcare events (e.g., birth and death) that affect census records.

7.2
AD Address

The Address data type is used to record postal addresses. They are modeled as a collection of geographic or political boundaries at various levels of detail and are used to deliver mail or packages. The CDA standard treats an address as an arbitrary list of address part elements (see Sect. 7.1 above) and text. This mixture of text and elements is called a *mixed content model* by the XML standard.

> **Mixed Models**
>
> *A mixed content model allows for an arbitrary collection of character data and subordinate elements to appear in another element.* It is used for elements containing text and other elements. In CDA the ED data type and <addr> and <name> elements use a mixed content model.
>
> The XML standard allows whitespace to be added between elements for readability, and parsers can ignore this whitespace. However, it is not possible to distinguish between the whitespace that has been added for readability and whitespace in the text in a mixed content model. All white space is significant because it represents text in the mixed content model.
>
> An example of mixed content appears below. It illustrates a an element containing child elements and text at the same level.
>
> ```
> <mixed>Text<child>Child 1</child> More Text
>   <child>Child 2</child>More Text
> </mixed>
> ```

According to the XML schema, each of the different parts of the <addr> element can appear as many times as necessary. However, it does not make sense for an address to have two <state> or <postalCode> elements. The same is true for several other elements. Almost all components should appear only once with the exception of the <streetAddressLine> or <deliveryAddressLine> element.

XML Encoding of Addresses

The preferred form for postal addresses in most systems appears in Fig. 7.1 below. This form of the address places the street address lines, city, state, postal code and country within XML elements that identify those address components.

```
<addr><streetAddressLine>17 Norroway
Ave</streetAddressLine>
<delimiter/><city>Randolph</city>, <state>MA</state>
<delimiter/><postalCode>02116</postalCode>
<delimiter/><country>USA</country>
</addr>
```

Fig. 7.1 Postal address preferred form

The ADDR data type also has a semantic property called the "formatted" property in the HL7 Abstract Data Types standard. This property represents the formatted form of the address for human reading. The formatted form appears with the proper line breaks and whitespace. This property is not transmitted because it can be reconstructed from the address parts contained within the ADDR data type according to local conventions. However, these address parts can appear in an arbitrary order according to those conventions. Transmitting addresses across boundaries where conventions are different can cause some difficulty between those systems if the addresses are to be used to communicate.

A solution to this problem is to transmit the data in the formatted form with the appropriate XML element markup to identify the address parts. This is done in the by including appropriate white space and delimiter tags in the <addr> element as shown above.

The <delimiter> element is used to identify formatting characters used inside the formatted address. Content inside this element is considered to be a delimiter of the address. If no characters appear inside the <delimiter> element, it is presumed to be a newline. Note the position of the <delimiter/> tag in the example above. It is used at the beginning of a line instead of at the end because any whitespace following the empty delimiter tag would be significant, including the terminal newline. The <delimiter> element cannot be used inside any other ADXP data element.

Figure 7.2 shows several uses of the <delimiter> element. The first use of this element wraps the new line between the street address and the city and is entirely equivalent to the last use of the element with no value. The <delimiter> element can also be used to identify other delimiting punctuation, as shown in the second use of the element in the example. In that case, it identifies the comma and space between the city and the state as delimiter characters. Note that the space between the state and the postal code in this example is not identified as a delimiter.

```
<addr>
17 Norroway Ave<delimiter>
</delimiter>Randolph<delimiter>, </delimiter>MA 02116<
delimiter/>
USA
</addr>
```

Fig. 7.2 Postal address with delimiters

It is entirely legal within the CDA standard to just enter the address completely as character data, as shown in Fig. 7.3. Systems assuming that the former example will be sent for an address may not capture the address at all because the elements for street address, city, state, et cetera, are not present.

```
<addr>
17 Norroway Ave
Randolph, MA 02116
USA
</addr>
```

Fig. 7.3 Postal address as text

The address data type can content more finely parsed addresses. Figure 7.4 below shows the same street address line used in Fig. 7.1 parsed at greater detail using some of the other XML elements that make up the set of parts defined by the ADXP data type.

```
<houseNumber>17</houseNumber>
<streetNameBase>Norroway</streetNameBase>
<streetNameType>Ave</streetNameType>
```

Fig. 7.4 Parsed street address line

You might think that having multiple levels of granularity for parsing a street address would allow for the following representation:

```
<addr>
   <streetAddressLine>
      <houseNumber>17</houseNumber>
      <streetNameBase>Norroway</streetNameBase>
      <streetNameType>Ave</streetNameType>
   </streetAddressLine>
   <city>Randolph</city>, <state>MA</state>
   <postalCode>02116</postalCode>
   <country>USA</country>
</addr>
```

Fig. 7.5 Overparsed postal address example

This is simply not supported.

7.3
Name Part

Names can be parsed into a collection of different parts, just like addresses. The Entity Name Part data type supports the representation of these different parts of a name. HL7 divides names up into three types, persons, organizations and other things including places. The names for people are parsed into prefixes, suffixes, given names, family names and delimiters. Organizational names can have prefixes or suffixes (e.g., Inc or BV) and delimiters. The names for places and things do not have different parts.

<delimiter>

The <delimiter> element marks the boundaries of delimiters in names.

<family>

The <family> element identifies components of the name that link a person to their parents.

<given>

The <family> element identifies components of a name that are given to a person. A person can have more than one given name. Each one is stored in the CDA document in the appropriate order.

<prefix>

The <prefix> element identifies components of names that have a strong connection to what follows it when the name is displayed normally (e.g., as one would when addressing mail or signing a document).

<suffix>

The <suffix> element identifies components of names that have a strong connection to what precedes it when displayed normally.

qualifier

The qualifier XML attribute describes the type of name part.

Table 7.1 Qualifier codes

Code	Name type	Description
LS	Legal status	Used on a suffix to indicate the legal status of an organization (e.g., Inc. or GmbH).
AC	academic	Used on a prefix or suffix to indicate an academic title (e.g., Dr. or M.D.)
NB	nobility	Used to identify a title of nobility (e.g., "von" in German).
PR	professional	Used to identify a professional association (e.g., FACEP or FPHIMSS).
VV	voorvoegsel	Identifies parts of a name that historically, but no longer, denote nobility (e.g., "van" in Dutch).
AD	adopted	Used to identify a name given at adoption.
BR	birth	Used to identify a name given at birth. May be used to identify the "maiden" name or for temporary names (e.g., baby boy).
SP	spouse	Used to identify a name assumed from the partner in a spousal relationship. Usually the spouse's family name. No inference about gender can be made from the existence of spouse names.
CL	callme	Used to identify the name that is preferred when a person is addressed directly.
IN	initial	Used to indicate that a name part is just an initial with no punctuation implied. May have more than one character (e.g., Th. for Thomas).
TITLE	title	Used to indicate that the prefix or a suffix is a title that applies to the whole name.

Contents of this table are drawn from the HL7 Vocabulary Standard with permission. Columns 1 and 2 come directly from the standard. Column 3 is the author's interpretation

7.4
EN Entity Name

Nouns are persons, places or things. Entity is simply another way to say noun. The Entity Name data type exists to supply names for various kinds of nouns. It supports the expression of names for organizations, persons, places or things in a single data type. The Entity Name is the data type from which organization name, person name and trivial name below are derived. This data type is only used in CDA to name drugs or other materials. The EN data type is a list of ENXP data elements, and like <addr> uses a mixed content model (see the sidebar on page 63) to contain the data.

While it is legal to use the <suffix>, <prefix>, <given> or <family> name parts in an Entity Name, these are rarely if ever used in a CDA document in items using the EN data

type. That is because drugs and other materials do not use names that are parsed in this fashion. HL7 choose to use Entity Name rather than the simpler Trivial Name data type (see Sect. 7.7 on page 72) for drugs and other materials because it was thought that drug and chemical names had as yet unidentified parts. For example, the legal names for drugs in the US and elsewhere include both the ingredient and the form of the drug. Since the entity name data type is the super type of the Trivial Name data type, it could readily be used to convey these name parts in future editions of CDA without changing the name of the data type used for medications. The data type of EN would of necessity change to incorporate the new part types, but the name would remain the same. This is being considered in the latest work by HL7 to accommodate different parts of names for some entities such as drugs. Many systems that read CDA documents will not know what to do when you supply the name of a drug or other material using any of the entity name parts.

use

The use attribute describes the use or representation of a name.

Table 7.2 Name uses

Code	Display name	Definition
C	License	Used only when the name recorded on a license or other document differs from the legal name.
I	Indigenous/Tribal	e.g. Chief Red Cloud
L	Legal	The legal name of the entity
P	pseudonym	A name that is used by a person or organization that differs from their legal name. This might refer to the name used by an organization doing business, or it may be another name that a person is known by. This is NOT commonly used to identify nicknames (see CALLME) under qualifier in ENXP above.
A	Artist/Stage	A name used by a performer when they perform, including a pen or stage name.
R	Religious	A name assumed upon assumption of a position in a religious order.
SRCH	search	A name used for searching.
PHON	phonetic	A phonetic spelling of the name.
SNDX	Soundex	A soundex code for a name.
ABC	Alphabetic	An alphabetic transcription for a name from another script (e.g., Japanese Romanji).
SYL	Syllabic	Transcription of a name into a syllabic script such as kana or hangul.
IDE	Ideographic	An ideographic representation of name (e.g., kanji)

Contents of this table are drawn from the HL7 Vocabulary Standard with permission. Columns 1 and 2 come directly from the standard. Column 3 is the author's interpretation.

<validTime> (See IVL_TS Interval of Time on Page 99)

Names are used for a period of time and may later be changed or discarded. The <validTime> element records the time interval over which the name is valid. The <validTime> element is of the IVL_TS data type described in the section on Dates below.

7.5
ON Organization Name

Organization names are a list of <prefix>, <suffix>, <delimiter> and text parts that represent the name of an organization. Two examples appear in the figures below.

```
<name>Health Level Seven International, Inc.</name>
```

Fig. 7.6 Organizational name example

```
<name>Health Level Seven International<delimiter>,
</delimiter><suffix qualifier='LS'>Inc.</suffix></name>
```

Fig. 7.7 Organizational name example with name parts

Suffixes typically appearing in organization names are abbreviations or acronyms such as LLC, Inc, or Gmbh. Organization names are typically represented in a CDA document without "parsing" the organization's name into separate parts.

Most CDA implementations do not use prefixes or suffixes with organization names.

7.6
PN Person Name

Person names are a list of <prefix>, <given>, <family>, <suffix> and <delimiter> elements and text. The PN data type is found in the <name> element of the <assignedPerson>, <associatedPerson>, <guardianPerson>, <informationRecipient>, <maintainingPerson>, <relatedPerson>, <playingEntity>, <specimenPlayingEntity> and <subject> elements. The PN data type is derived from the EN data type and so also supports the use attribute and the <validTime> element of that data type.

A sample represent of the <name> element is shown in below for my name.

```
<name><prefix>Mr.</prefix> <given>Keith</given> <given
qualifier='initial'>W.</given> <family>Boone</family>
</name>
```

Fig. 7.8 A <name> with sub-elements

Because the PN data type is a restriction of the EN data type, it also has a mixed content model (see the sidebar on page 63). This means that the <name> element can simply contain the text representation of the person's name with no other subordinate elements as shown in the figure below.

```
<name>Mr. Keith W. Boone</name>
```

Fig. 7.9 A <name> without sub-elements

Like the AD data type, the PN data type has a formatted form that is not transmitted in the exchange. Again I recommend transmission of the name in the appropriate order based on local conventions in effect. In this way the formatted property can be easily determined from the exchanged information found in the CDA document.

The order and number of the <name> components and size of the text content is not prescribed by the XML ITS. This is because various cultures structure names differently. Some cultures place the family name first, followed by the given name, while others (such as my own) place them in the opposite order. Other cultures commonly use several family names to effectively create an ancestral genealogy in the family name.

Many cultures provide a person with two or more given names. My youngest daughter has three given names, one first and two middle names. Few information systems are able to correctly store the structure of her name. They will often store her two middle names together in one field.

If she chose after marriage to exchange her middle names for her maiden name, she would then have one given name and two family names. She could also choose to preserve her middle names, and take on her husband's family name in addition to her own family name, and may or may not hyphenate the family name as her last name. She would then have three given names and two family names. If she hyphenated her family name, it might be represented in a single <family> name element with the embedded hyphen, or as two separate <family> name elements with an intervening <delimiter> containing the hyphen.

CDA implementations should carefully consider how names are both represented in an exchange and stored in an information system. In addition to name structure and the various name parts, consideration must also be given to character set limitations.

Inversion

Names are commonly inverted when presented by information systems to make it easier to find people. This is often done in directories in regions where the family name comes last (as it does in many Western cultures). When names are inverted, the prefix is usually put after the first part of the name instead of before it (e.g., Boone, Keith W. Mr.).

I know of no CDA implementations that transmit names in the inverted form, but I have received a few questions about its use. While the XML ITS comments on inversion, it neither prohibits nor promotes its use. I do not recommend transmitting names in a CDA document in inverted form. There is no way to indicate that the name was inverted in the CDA, and thus no way to determine the proper order.

Character Set Considerations

Because the CDA standard uses XML, any legal Unicode character can appear in a name in a CDA document. However, many information systems storing a person's name are limited to character sets that do not support the full range of expression of Unicode. Well designed systems will normalize characters that cannot be represented using an appropriate substitute. For example, systems that support only the US ASCII encoding might represent accented characters using their unaccented forms. Note that some characters that appear to be "accented" are treated as distinct characters in different languages. Systems performing normalization should process all possible representations.

Many different character presentations have more than one way of being represented in Unicode. Unicode contains special characters that change the presentation of the preceding character by adding a *diacritical mark*. A diacritical is a mark added to a character to indicate a change in its pronunciation. Accent marks are just one type of diacritical mark. These are known as combining characters. Information systems that perform character normalization should recognize the various Unicode representations of the same character presentation. The Unicode Technical Report #15 Unicode Normalization Forms [1] describes a method known as Normalization form C that can be used to create a canonical form for Unicode text that eliminates these variations.

Information System Considerations

Names are used in healthcare to assist in the unique identification of patients, providers and related persons. Precision in the representation of the structure of the name in every last detail is less important than the ability of these systems to use the name to find the person it identifies. Information systems are often designed to address variations in names according to local requirements. In the Western world, many information systems divide names up into as many as seven distinct parts. These name parts include the honorific or prefix, first name, middle name, last name, suffix, degree, and sometimes maiden name. These information systems typically support only one part of each type.

The table below shows conventions that can be used to map between these name parts and the elements used in CDA.

Table 7.3 Name Part mapping to CDA

Name Part	CDA element
Honorific	`<prefix>`
First Name	`<given>`
Middle Name	`<given>`
Maiden Name	`<family qualifier='BR'>`
Last Name	`<family>`
Suffix	`<suffix>`
Degree	`<suffix qualifier='AC'>`

Using these conventions should provide the appropriate recall characteristics needed to identify different persons. Note that the name alone is insufficient to uniquely identify an individual. My youngest daughter's first and last names are the same as my wife, an issue that typically causes delay when we check in at the airport. Of course their birthdates are quite distinct, but even that is not enough in all situations. One of my mentors in college was an identical twin who shared not only a family name and birth date with his brother, but also the first two given names. The distinction between these two was in their third given name.

7.7
TN Trivial Name

The names of places and things are considered to be trivial names because they are not parsed into different parts like names of people or organizations.

7.8
II Instance Identifier

The II data type is used to identify different instances of a kind of thing. This data type is used extensively in the CDA specification to identify persons, places, things, actions, roles, et cetera. The II data type most commonly appears in the `<id>` elements found in the CDA schema. It is also used by the `<setId>`, `<templateId>` and `<typeId>` elements.

In some cases, the CDA standard allows a collection (a set) of identifiers to be used for something. This is because the same thing may be know by different organizations using different identifiers. The most common case is for the placer and filler order numbers for an order. Another common case is when preexisting identifiers get re-used to identify a person in a particular role (e.g., a license or DEA number for a healthcare provider).

root

Every element using the II data must have a root attribute that uniquely identifies the set of identifiers which it may contain. This is known as the namespace of the identifier. The namespace is simply a named set of things.

The root XML attribute often indicates the organization that assigned the identifier, otherwise known as its assigning authority. In some cases the root attribute simple identifies a universe containing only one thing. In these cases it does not represent an assigning authority; it is simply a universal identifier. The root attribute is required in all instances of this type that do not contain an exceptional value (e.g., an unknown).

The root attribute must be stored as either an ISO Object Identifier (OID) or a Universal Identifier (UUID). The former are preferred by HL7 specifications and implementation guides (see [DT§2.15] which states: UUIDs are **not** the preferred identifier scheme for use as HL7 UIDs.)

UUIDs are also known as GUIDs (Globally Unique Identifiers) due to the use of this acronym by a common operating system vendor. Neither GUID nor UUID should be confused with UID, which is a common acronym used by the DICOM standard to refer to an OID.

The value of the root attribute is an *opaque* string. From an engineering perspective, something that is opaque cannot be looked into. Don't try. You may think you see something, but your vision is likely obscured. That means that it can be used for tests of equality, but that you should not try to interpret its structure. It does not mean that you may not use a particular structure when you create OIDs or UUIDs for objects, only that you should not make any assumptions about the syntax of that structure when you use it.

OID Representation

In HL7 specifications an OID is represented as a sequence of non-negative integers separated by periods. They look like an IP address on steroids. For example, the OID for HL7 appears as 2.16.840.1.113883. Note that there are no leading zeros in the representation of the numeric portions. HL7 provides a publically available OID registry from which anyone (even non-members) can obtain an OID for their own use or look up OIDs used or assigned to others. This is available at http://www.hl7.org/oid/index.cfm.

Stupid Geek Tricks

Try this trick. Take the trouble to remember this OID: 2.16.840.1.113883, and the last parts of OIDs that matter to you, such as 5.4 = HL7 ActCode, 6.1 = LOINC, 6.88 = RxNORM, 6.96 = SNOMED CT, 6.103 ICD-9-CM Diagnoses and 6.104 = ICD-9-CM Procedures. You can recite OIDs off the top of your head and amaze your friends.

The HL7 Implementation Guide for Unique Object Identifiers informative specification is available from the HL7 website at http://www.hl7.org and provides a great deal of information about how to use OIDs inside CDA documents.

Each number in an OID is of unlimited length. Practical considerations indicate that OIDs components should be limited to values between 1 and 2^{31}-1 (about 2 billion values) because some application libraries use arrays of integers to store OID values (Inappropriately I might add given the formal definition of an OID.) OIDs should be less than 64 characters in length to support exchange of them in information systems using other standards (such as DICOM) that are limited to that length.

UUID Representation

UUIDs appear in the form ########-####-####-####-############ where each # symbol is a single hexadecimal digit (in upper case [DT§2.5.1]).

RFC 4122 [2] describes the syntax more formally in the production for UUID. Several database applications assign a UUID to rows of tables. This makes the UUID form particularly convenient for use in identifying objects, as there is a one to one correspondence between the identifier of a thing in a CDA document and an identifier associated with its storage in an information retrieval system.

ITU-T X.667 [3] describes a translation of a UUID into an OID. The UUID is first converted to an integer according to the rules found in section 6.3, and that integer is then appended to the string 2.25. to create the OID representation. Note that this creates an OID which contains an integer component larger than 32 bits in length.

extension

The extension attribute of the II data type uniquely identifies an instance of a thing contained within namespace identified by the root attribute. It is used when the root alone is insufficient to uniquely identify something. The extension attribute is commonly used with identifiers that are externally assigned, for example, for visits, accounts, medical record numbers, and identifiers issued by governments for people and organizations.

displayable

The displayable attribute indicates whether the identifier stored is intended to be displayed to humans for data entry. As a general rule identifiers which do not contain an extension attribute will not be useful for human consumption. Identifiers which do contain an extension attribute may be suitable for human consumption, but you cannot always make that assumption. Many rather long identifiers would not be readily accessible for human use. This often includes identifiers generated for producing bar codes. This attribute is advisory, as there may be certain situations where an identifier may need to be displayed regardless of its complexity.

assigningAuthorityName

The `assigningAuthorityName` attribute provides a human readable name for the assigning authority associated with an identifier. This attribute is provided purely for convenience and has no computed semantic interpretation. It is rather hard to remember which universe of identifiers each OID represents. This attribute makes it possible to provide a human readable interpretation for those that have not mastered stupid geek tricks.

7.9
TEL Telecommunications Address

A telecommunications address or endpoint specifies how to contact someone or something using telecommunications equipment. That includes the telephone, a fax machine, e-mail, the web, instant messaging, et cetera. All telecommunications addresses can be represented by a URI. The TEL data type is used in the `<telecom>` elements found in various entities and roles, and also appears in the `<reference>` element used by the ED data type (see page 49).

value

The `value` attribute of a `<telecom>` data element provides the URI identifying the communications endpoint. Different types of endpoints are represented by URI forms using different URI schemes. The scheme used indicates the type of communications endpoint.

Usually when a data element uses the `nullFlavor` XML attribute, other attributes (such as `value`) are not permitted in the representation. The TEL data type doesn't work that way. That is because the type of endpoint and the endpoint location are combined into one field. It would be difficult to communicate an unknown telephone or e-mail address if you did not at least indicate the type of URL.

So, to indicate an unknown telephone number, e-mail address, instant messaging, or web address, you could use the forms shown below, but it may not be supported as a legal URL in your XML parser.

```
<!-- an unknown telephone number -->
<telecom nullFlavor='UNK' value='tel:'/>
<!-- an unknown e-mail address -->
<telecom nullFlavor='UNK' value='mailto:'/>
<!-- an unknown instant messaging address -->
<telecom nullFlavor='UNK' value='im:'/>
<!-- an unknown website -->
<telecom nullFlavor='UNK' value='http:'/>
```

Fig. 7.10 Unknown telecommunications addresses

Newer releases of the data type specifications address separate the type of communications from the address and will be supported in the next release of CDA.

Telephone and Fax

Telephones and fax equipment can be represented using the `tel:` URI schemes defined in RFC 3966 which replaced the earlier RFC 2806 used in the XML ITS. Technically, the CDA Standards relies on a specific version of the XML ITS, which in turn relies on RFC 2086, not RFC 3966. However, compatibility with both RFCs is desirable and readily achieved. Both of these RFCs define the `tel:` URI scheme as being composed of a global phone number or a local phone number and context, followed by a number of dialing parameters. The global number starts with a plus (+) symbol and is followed by the country code and national phone number. The local number starts with a digit and also contains a context parameter that gives the local context. The local context is represented using the global dialing digits.

Since a local phone number must include a context containing the global dialing digits, there is no reason to support both forms. A refinement of RFC 3966 format is often used to exchange phone numbers. This is shown in the figure below.

```
telephone-url = 'tel:' global-phone-number [extension]
global-phone-number = '+' phone-number
phone-number = digits
digits = phonedigit | digits phonedigit
phonedigit = DIGIT | visual-separator
extension = ';ext=' digits
visual-separator = '-' | '.' | '(' | ')'
```

Fig. 7.11 Telephone URI refinement

This refinement prohibits the use of local numbers, and requires extensions to appear using the RFC 3966 format. It also eliminates other dialing parameters which Healthcare Information Systems would be unlikely to use.

The examples below show the tel: URL syntax in use, with and without an extension.

```
<telecom value='tel:+1(999)999-9999;ext=99999'/>
<telecom value='tel:+1(999)999-9999'/>
```

Fig. 7.12 Example use of the tel: URL format

Note that the examples below are incorrect, because they do not include the country code.

```
<telecom value='tel:(999)999-9999;ext=99999'/>
<telecom value='tel:(999)999-9999'/>
```

Fig. 7.13 Incorrect use of the tel: URL

Visual separators (parenthesis, periods and hyphens) in phone numbers are used as an aid to memorization, and have no semantic meaning in the telephone number URI. These characters should be ignored when comparing two telephone number URIs.

RFC 2806 also included a fax: URL scheme that distinguished a voice line from a fax line, but this distinction was removed in the updated RFC 3966. The next release of the HL7 data types will support a new attribute on the TEL data type to list connection capabilities (voice, fax, data, teletype and short message service). That data type will be supported in CDA Release 3.

The extension parameter was not formally defined in RFC 2806, but that RFC did allow for arbitrary parameters to be added to the URI, which makes this restricted specification conform to both RFCs. This specification for phone numbers has been adopted in the IHE Patient Care Coordination Technical Framework.

E-mail

E-mail addresses are represented using the `mailto:` URI scheme defined in RFC 2368. Technically, more than one e-mail address is permitted in the `mailto:` URI scheme and additional parameters describing the subject line and body of the message may also be present. CDA Implementations using this scheme to send e-mail addresses usually do not send anything other than a single e-mail address following the `mailto:` URI scheme identifiers. While this is a commonly adopted convention in exchanges of CDA documents it is often implied and not made a specific requirement.

Web Sites

Web site addresses are formatted using the `http:` and `https:` URI formats which are described in RFC 2396.

Instant Messaging

Instant messaging URIs should use the im: URI scheme defined in RFC 3860. This RFC borrows heavily from the mailto: URI scheme. To represent my instant messaging address in the CDA document you would use `<telecom value='im:kwboone@skype.com'/>`.

Like e-mail addresses, instant messaging addresses support additional parameters that are not likely to be needed in a CDA document.

The im: URI scheme is not commonly recognized by many applications that parse URIs. Most instant messaging services use proprietary protocols that cannot be used outside of a single messaging domain.

Texting and Short Messaging Service (SMS)

Most phone services supporting text messaging also support an e-mail address to which SMS messages can be sent, but other non-telephone devices also accept short messages. The sms: URI scheme specified in RFC 5724 combines telephone numbers from the tel: URI with the syntax of the mailto: URI to specify the message body and other parameters. Again, these additional parameters are not typically needed to exchange the text messaging number.

use

The use attribute provides codes from the table below describing the type of communications endpoint. There is some overlap between some of these codes and the type of URL that is used. For example, pagers typically support the short messaging service.

Table 7.4 Codes for the use attribute

Code	Display name	Comments
H	home address	A personal or home phone, e-mail address, or other personal device.
HP	primary home	The usual address used to reach a person after business hours.
HV	vacation home	The address used to reach a person during vacations.
WP	work place	A phone number, e-mail address, et cetera associated with a person's employment.
DIR	Direct	A direct line accessing a person.
PUB	Public	A general business number which may reach a receptionist, automated system or other access point before the intended party.
BAD	bad address	Used to identify an address known to be invalid.
TMP	temporary address	A temporary communications address (see Sect. 7.9.3)
AS	answering service	A telephone number used to leave messages.
EC	emergency contact	A phone number explicitly to be used in case of emergencies.
MC	mobile contact	A cell phone or other mobile communications device.
PG	pager	A pager or other device uses to leave short messages.

Contents of this table are drawn from the HL7 Vocabulary Standard with permission. Columns 1 and 2 come directly from the standard. Column 3 is the author's interpretation.

<useablePeriod> (See GTS General Timing Specification on Page 103)

The `<useablePeriod>` element describes the time over which the communication address is available. This element uses the GTS data type described on page 103. Pragmatically, few systems are capable of interpreting so broad as specification as GTS. CDA implementations which use this element should constrain the use of this element to a more limited data type like IVL_TS or PIVL_TS. Because the `<usablePeriod>` element is of the GTS data type, it may appear more than once.

Summary

- Names and addresses can mix text and XML elements.
- There are more than 25 different parts that can be used for an address, but only 6 are commonly used.
- Name parts can appear in just about any order.
- Identifiers have one part that ensures uniqueness, found in the `root` XML attribute, and an optional part found in the `extension` XML attribute that can be used to represent the rest of the identifier when necessary.
- ISO Object Identifiers (OIDs) are the preferred form for representing the root XML attribute, but Universally Unique Identifiers (UUIDs) are also permitted.
- Telecommunications addresses of all types are represented using URLs.
- You cannot represent an "unknown" telecommunications address of a specific type without a trading partner agreement on the meaning of an unknown telecommunications address.

Questions

1. What is a mixed model and why is it important in a discussion of HL7 data types for names and addresses?
2. What element should be used to represent the "PO BOX 1" part of an address in a CDA `<addr>` element? Where else might you find this data? Why?
3. How would you indicate that a `<name>` element contains a person's legal name?
4. How might you document character set issues in an interface specification?
5. How would you identify a patient's home e-mail address?

Research Questions

1. How many different parts of an address are defined in the HL7 Data Types specification? Entity name parts?

2. What would you add to the following XML to represent that 999 is the patient's medical record number? How would this be different if it was a physician's national provider identifier? What tools might you use to locate the right answers to these questions?

```
<id extension='999'/>
```

References

1. Unicode Technical Report #15 Unicode Normalization Forms, November 11, 1999, The Unicode Consortium. Available on the web at http://www.unicode.org/reports/tr15/tr15-18.html
2. RFC 4122 A Universally Unique IDentifier (UUID) URN Namespace, Part 3, July 2005, Internet Engineering Task Force. Available from the web at http://www.ietf.org/rfc/rfc4122.txt
3. ITU-T X.667 Information technology – Open Systems Interconnection – Procedures for the operation of OSI Registration Authorities: Generation and registration of Universally Unique Identifiers (UUIDs) and their use as ASN.1 object identifier components, Section 6.3 and Section 7, September 2004, ITU-T. Available on the web at http://www.itu.int/ITU-T/study-groups/com17/oid/X.667-E.pdf

Codes and Vocabularies

8

This chapter appears before the introduction of the various data types used to support coding because of the importance of codes in the CDA™ (and HL7 Version 3 standards in general).

Vocabulary is an important component in the HL7 Reference Information Model. The HL7 Version 3 Reference Information Model is often described as a language for communicating about healthcare. If the RIM is the language, the codes that are used by Version 3 standards are the words that give this language an extensible meaning in the ever advancing world of healthcare. New codes are introduced regularly as important new ideas, diseases and treatments are discovered. Codes are used extensively in CDA to communicate about problems, medications, allergies, procedures, and a host of other concepts.

The use of codes to communicate between software applications goes back to the very first computer systems. The very instructions that they execute are simply codes that tell the computer what to do. Codes are short, and have a very well defined meaning. Narrative text requires a lot more care to avoid ambiguity.

Coding systems are like any other standard. For any given purpose there are usually several to chose from. Sometimes the choice of codes are easily made because certain sets of codes are required by law, and in other cases, a lot more debate and discussion is needed.

8.1
Concepts

A noun is a person, place, thing or idea. Codes are used to identify these various concepts. The concept may be very discrete, as in a specific medication in specific packaging with a given set of active ingredients, or it may be broad, describing a particular class of disorders.

Coding systems use different ways to define the boundaries of the concepts represented by a particular code.

- The HL7 Version 3 vocabularies provide a human readable definition for the concepts that they represent.
- ICD-9-CM and ICD-10-CM provide a collection of terms that can be used to determine whether concept is included or excluded from the idea represented by a particular code.

K.W. Boone, *The CDA™ Book*,
DOI: 10.1007/978-0-85729-336-7_8, © Springer-Verlag London Limited 2011

- LOINC describes laboratory tests by describing the (usually chemical) component being measured, the substance being analyzed, data type of the measurement produced, the specific laboratory method used to generate the result, and a number of other attributes to completely define a code.
- SNOMED CT provides a number of preferred and alternative terms (synonyms) for a concept, and also uses the position of the concept in the code hierarchy to define the meaning of the concept.
- Finally, UCUM uses the rules of mathematics to define the meaning of its coded concepts.

8.2
Codes

A code identifies a unique concept in a coding system. Multiple codes may represent the same concept, but this is rarely used in coding systems.

Codes can be opaque identifiers, meaning that the code value itself has no human interpretable structure. SNOMED CT and UMLS use opaque identifiers. These types of coding systems require some sort of human interface to select appropriate codes for a concept. Some organizations develop interface vocabularies for these coding systems. These provide readily understood and easily remembered phrases to locate codes.

Codes can also have an interpretable structure. The ICD-9-CM and ICD-10-CM coding systems are organized hierarchically. The code has different recognizable chunks that make it easy for humans to remember code values. Human coders can often code several clinical documents using ICD-9-CM without needing to look up any codes because of the structure of the code system. The structure of the coding system is the human interface into it.

8.3
Coding Systems

A coding system is a collection of codes. Coding systems can be simple lists of terms that are not explicitly related to each other (e.g., LOINC), or they can be organized in a hierarchy (e.g., ICD-9-CM and ICD-10-CM), or through a variety of different relationships (e.g., SNOMED CT).

The numbers of concepts that coding system can represent may be finite in length (e.g., LOINC and ICD-9-CM), or have infinite length via post-coordination (e.g., SNOMED CT) or code construction rules (e.g., UCUM).

Coding Systems can have multiple versions. Best practice for coding indicates that a code is never reused in different versions to represent different concepts, but this is not always adhered to in all coding systems (e.g., ICD-9-CM). For coding systems such as these, sending the coding system version is important in the communication, since it could not otherwise be clear which definition of a code was being used.

Each code in a coding system identifies a unique concept. A code can be atomic, representing a single simple concept or it can represent a complex concept that is made up of smaller concepts.

8.4
Pre- and Post-coordination

When a single code represents a composition of concepts it is using what is known as pre-coordination. In other cases, several codes may be used together in controlled ways to represent a composition of concepts. This type of coding is called post-coordination. Coding systems can include pre-coordinated concepts with distinct codes, or they can support post-coordination of several codes to represent a complex concept, or they can do both.

Some coding systems are developed intentionally to support the use of composition using different codes to describe various attributes of a concept. SNOMED CT is one example of a coding system that supports post-coordination. These coding systems may also contain pre-coordinated concepts to express a complex post-coordinated concept. CDA implementations that use these code systems should be prepared to process both representations of the concept. CDA implementations should also consider whether business rules of the exchange should allow or prohibit the use of these alternate representations. The HL7 TERMINFO specification provides guidance on the use of post-coordinated SNOMED CT concepts.

Other commonly used coding systems specify all details of a concept in a single code, and may merge several simpler concepts together under a single code. For example, the code for Diabetes with Renal Failure in ICD-9-CM merges these two separate concepts under one code. This is an example of pre-coordination.

8.5
Value Sets

A value set is a collection of codes from possibly more than one coding system representing a set of (usually) distinct concepts. Value Sets can represent subsets of a coding system used for a specific purpose, and are commonly used as a way to constrain the legal values appearing in an implementation guide.

An extensional value set is defined by enumerating each code found in it. Intentional value sets are defined by providing the rules (an algorithm) to determine whether a code is a member of the set. Value sets can have subsets which are also value sets, and these can also be defined intentionally or extensionally.

Intentional Value sets can be dynamic, which means that the set of values produced by it can vary as the underlying code system(s) are updated, or they can be static, using a fixed code system version. Extensional value sets are always static.

Value sets should be drawn from a single code system where possible. Value sets used by HL7 specifications, including CDA, are identified by a unique identifier called an OID (see OID Representation on page 73) and can have multiple versions.

Summary

- Coding is a fundamental feature of the HL7 Reference Information Model.
- Codes represent concepts.
- A coding system is a collection of codes which identify discrete concepts that is maintained by an organization.
- The use of post-coordination allows complex concepts to be described using simpler concepts.
- Coding systems can represent finite or infinite sets of concepts.
- A value set is a set of codes, possibly from multiple code systems, that can be defined by listing the codes in it, or by describing algorithmically what codes should be present.

Questions

1. How does a value set differ from a coding system? How are they similar?
2. Can the same code represent two different concepts in a coding system?
3. Can the same concept be represented by two different codes in a coding system?
4. True or false: A single code representing the conjunction of two simpler concepts uses post-coordination.

Research Questions

1. Describe two different codes that represent the same concept in a coding system. Why are these two different codes present in the coding system?
2. Describe two different concepts that are represented by the same code in a coding system. Why do these two different concepts use the same code? How would you distinguish between the two?

Codes

9

Codes represent distinct concepts in a coding system, also called a terminology or vocabulary. All coded representations in HL7 derive from the Concept Descriptor (CD) data type described in more detail below.

The data types that follow use the same components as the CD data type. These components are only described once under the CD data type. The table below shows which of these components are allowed for each data type.

Table 9.1 Components used by data type

	CD	CE	CV	CO	CS
code	✓	✓	✓	✓	✓
displayName	✓	✓	✓	✓	
codeSystem	✓	✓	✓	✓	
codeSystemName	✓	✓	✓	✓	
codeSystemVersion	✓	✓	✓	✓	
<originalText>	✓	✓	✓	✓	
<translation>	✓	✓			
<qualifier>	✓				

Coded data types are conceptually similar to the II data type. The `codeSystem` attribute indentifies a set (or namespace) of concepts just as the `root` attribute of the II data type identifies a set (or namespace) of identifiers. The `code` attribute identifies a specific concept within that set just as the `extension` attribute identifies a specific instance of an identifier within the II data type. These data type vary from the II data type in that the `codeSystem` attribute must always be an OID and may not be a UUID, and must always be present.

The `code` and `codeSystem` attributes are required for non-exceptional values. Other XML attributes are optional. The XML attributes are usually not allowed when the coded data type contains an exceptional value (e.g., `nullFlavor='UNK'`). When `nullFlavor` takes on the value of OTH, the `codeSystem` attribute is required to be present to indicate which coding system the value could not be coded in.

The `<originalText>`, `<translation>`, and `<qualifier>` elements are always permitted.

K.W. Boone, *The CDA™ Book*,
DOI: 10.1007/978-0-85729-336-7_9, © Springer-Verlag London Limited 2011

9.1
CD Concept Descriptor

The concept descriptor data type is the most complex of the coded data types. In addition to several attributes describing the code, it can contain a reference to the original text that was encoded in the `<originalText>` element, additional codes that further qualify the original code in the `<qualifier>` element, and translations of the original code to other code systems in the `<translation>` element.

code

The `code` attribute contains the identifier of the concept being represented by the coding system. This is a string value.

displayName

The `displayName` XML attribute provides a human readable name for the code. This attribute carries no computable semantics and is simply provided as an aid for human interpretation. I recommend that CDA™ implementations include the `displayName` XML attribute since it dramatically simplifies debugging.
In a CDA document, the `displayName` should normally appear in the same language as the document is written in (see `languageCode` under Other document descriptors on page 136).

codeSystem

The `codeSystem` XML attribute contains an OID (see OID Representation on page 73) that identifies the coding system being used. The OID identifies the assigning authority of the code.
   Some terminologies have more than one code value representing the same concept, to support coding using legacy code values. For example, SNOMED CT also lists the legacy Read and SNOMED International codes used for existing SNOMED CT concepts. Technically these are different coding systems and so should not use the same OID for the preferred codes of the terminology.

codeSystemName

The `codeSystemName` XML attribute provides a human readable name for the code system. This attribute carries no computable semantics and is simply provided as an aid for human interpretation. I recommend that CDA implementations include the `codeSystemName` attribute since it dramatically simplifies debugging and avoids the need to perform stupid geek tricks (see footnote at the bottom of page 73). In a CDA document, the codeSystemName should normally appear in the same language as the document is written in (see languageCode under Other Document Descriptors on page 136).

codeSystemVersion

The codeSystemVersion XML attribute identifiers the version of the coded vocabulary used. This attribute is either the official version number as given by the maintaining party or when no version number is assigned, the release date. There are many different ways to represent release date, but I would recommend the use of the YYYYMMDD format to represent dates.

This attribute can be vital in interpreting information when a coding system reuses codes previously assigned (as was done for some ICD-9-CM codes several years back). Note, most coding systems today do not reassign codes (it's not a best practice).

<originalText> (See ED Encapsulated Data on Page 49)

The <originalText> element contains the original text that was coded. This text may be included by reference or by value. Figure 9.1 below shows the use of the <originalText> element where the text content is contained by reference. The following figure shows the how the <orginalText> element would be written to contain the text by value. Typically the original text used for coding appears in the CDA document and should be included by reference instead of by value. This also allows style sheets that render CDA documents to linked coded values in the narrative portion of the document to the machine readable code. For more information see the ED data type on page 49.

```
<section>
   <text>… patient had a <content ID='ref'>heart
attack</content>…</text>
   <entry>         …
      <code   code='410.9'
              displayName='myocardial infarction'
              codeSystem='2.16.840.1.113883.6.103'
              codeSystemName='ICD-9-CM'>
   <originalText><reference
value='#ref'/></originalText>
      </code>
   </entry>
</section>
```

Fig. 9.1 <originalText> cited by reference

```
    ...
<originalText>Heart Attack</originalText>
    ...
```

Fig. 9.2 `<originalText>` contained by value

`<qualifier>` (LIST_CR)

The `<qualifier>` element allows a code to be stored compositionally. It contains a list of one or more concept roles that provide more information about the concept being encoded. Qualifiers are used with coding systems like SNOMED CT which allow codes to be composed of other codes in a post-coordinated fashion. Figure 9.3 below shows an example using the `<qualifier>` element to indicate the location (finding site) of a myocardial infarction.

```
<code code='22298006'
      displayName='myocardial infarction'
      codeSystem='2.16.840.1.113883.6.96'
      codeSystemName='SNOMED CT'>
   <qualifier>
      <name code='363698007' displayName='finding site'
          codeSystem='2.16.840.1.113883.6.96'/>
      <value code='73050001'
          displayName='anterolateral region'
          codeSystem='2.16.840.1.113883.6.96'/>
   </qualifier>
</code>
```

Fig. 9.3 A `<qualifer>` example

The HL7 Abstract Data Types specification explains that `<qualifier>` elements modify the coded concept. It is better to say that `<qualifier>` elements provide more information about the concept. You would not for example, negate the original concept using a qualifier, or refine it to a degree that it was no longer an instance of the original concept being qualified. Note that the `<qualifier>` element may not be used with a concept from a code system that does not support composition.

`<name>` (See Sect. 9.3 Below)

The `<name>` element contains the name of the role played by the qualifier. This can be text, in which case it is stored under the `<originalText>` component of the `<name>` element, or it can be a coded value, in which case the `<name>` element will have a code and codeSystem attribute (and may also include an `<originalText>` element).

<value> (See Sect. 9.1 Above)

The <value> element contains the coded value describing the additional qualifier.

inverted

The inverted attribute is used on the qualifier to indicate that the direction of the role relationship is inverted. The default value of this attribute is false.

Suppose a coding system describes a condition (e.g., liver malfunction), a disease (hepatitis C), and a relationship between them (e.g., caused by). A coded concept using these three could use the code for *liver malfunction*, with a qualifier that had a name of *caused by*, and a value of *hepatitis C*.

```
<code code='liver malfunction' codeSystem='…'>
    <qualifer inverted='false'>
        <name code='caused by' codeSystem='…'/>
        <value code='hepatitis C' codeSystem='…'/>
    </qualifier>
</code>
```

Fig. 9.4 Uninverted qualifier

However, this could also be coded using the code for *hepatitis C* with a qualifier name of *caused by*, and a value of *liver malfunction*, with the inverted attribute set to true on the <qualifier> element.

```
<code code='hepatitis C' codeSystem='…'>
    <qualifer inverted='true'>
        <name code='caused by' codeSystem='…'/>
        <value code='liver malfunction' codeSystem='…'/>
    </qualifier>
</code>
```

Fig. 9.5 Inverted qualifier

This attribute is rarely used because the few code systems that support inversion usually contain reciprocal pairs of role names (e.g., causes and caused by). However, it does mean that CDA applications using post-coordinated coding using the CD data type should be able to recognize multiple representations of a concept including the use of the inverted attribute.

\<translation\> (SET_CD)

The \<translation\> element is used to store translations of a coded concept from one coding system using codes from another coding system. Multiple \<translation\> elements may be provided for a single coded concept. Translations contain approximate equivalences between the two coded concepts, and it should not be assumed that the same two concepts are identical.

```
<code code='410.9' displayName='myocardial infarction'
      codeSystem='2.16.840.1.113883.6.103'
      codeSystemName='ICD-9-CM'>
  <translation code='22298006'
      codeSystem='2.16.840.1.113883.6.96'
      codeSystemName='SNOMED CT'/>
</code>
```

Fig. 9.6 \<translation\> example

The definition of the \<translation\> element makes it clear that the direction of the translation is from the code specified in the coded concept to the code specified in the \<translation\> element, and provides no mechanism to alter the direction of the translation. This implication of coding and translation order is sometimes ignored in exchange specifications that require concepts to be exchanged using a specific coding system. Information systems participating in the exchange may identify the concept in one coding system (e.g., ICD-9-CM), but be required to exchange it in another (e.g., SNOMED CT) in the \<code\> element. Because of the approximate nature of translations, this is not seen as a major issue. The Release 2 Data Types specification addresses this issue and will be used in CDA Release 3.

The benefit of using translation is that it permits systems to use concepts that they are familiar with. For example, the codeSystem required for exchange of the medication code could be specified to be RxNORM, but if the sender and receiver both support the same proprietary vocabulary system, sending the proprietary code in a \<translation\> element may provide a more precise exchange of information.

9.2
CE Coded with Equivalents

The CE data type is used to exchange coded concepts that are not permitted to contain qualifiers and so do not allow for codes to be created compositionally using post-coordination. There are some questions about when you might use CE instead of CD. The simple answer would be to use CE only if the coding system selected for the exchange does not support post-coordination.

9.3
CV Coded Value

The CV data type derives from the CE data type. It is used when only an unqualified coded concept without translations is desired in an exchange. The CV data type is used for example in the <name> element of a <qualifier> because:

1. There is no need for a translation of the qualifier name into another coding system because qualifiers only work in the coding in which they are designed, and
2. The qualifier name is not itself a complex concept that needs to be built compositionally from other coded concepts.

9.4
CO Coded Ordinal

The CO data type derives from the CV data type. It has the additional property that the various codes are ordered. Codes may be used to describe various stages of disease, where each stage is more advanced than another. The use of the CO data type implies an ordering among these codes. Note that use of this data type does not mean that the order can be determined by application software without some knowledge of the coding system in use. The code attribute need not be numeric.

Even when the code attribute is numeric, software applications should not assume that these numbers do anything other than order the codes. For example, consider a disease such as cancer which is often described as being at Stage I, Stage II, Stage III, or Stage IV. It is meaningless to subtract Stage II from Stage IV or to relate the differences between these two stages to the differences between Stage I and Stage III.

9.5
CS Coded Simple

The CS data type is used to convey codes that have a fixed value for codeSystem. It is used in the CDA specification for coded values where there is only one choice for the codeSystem according to the standard.

It is used in the <realmCode>, <languageCode>, <statusCode> and <signatureCode> elements in the CDA specification.

```
<realmCode code='US'/>
<languageCode code='en-US'/>
<statusCode code='completed'/>
<signatureCode code='S'/>
```

Fig. 9.7 CS examples

The CS data type should not be used elsewhere in the CDA where a fixed vocabulary has not been defined by the CDA standard itself. Do not be tempted to use this for example in a `<value>` element in an `<observation>`.

Summary

- Codes identify unique concepts in a space of concepts defined by a coding system.
- HL7 identifies coding systems using an OID.
- The CD data type represents a concept, which can have a code in a coding system, the original text describing the concept, a number of codes refining the original concept (called qualifiers), and translations to other coding systems.
- All of the different coded data types derive from the Concept Descriptor (CD) data type.

Questions

1. Is the following a legal representation of a Concept Descriptor (CD) data type?

```
<code nullFlavor='OTH'>
    <originalText>Heart Attack</originalText>
</code>
```

2. What two attributes of the CD data type are optional and why would you use them in an implementation?
3. Is this a legal representation of a Concept Descriptor when #ref1 points to text containing the word "Heart Attack".

```
<text>… The patient suffered from a <content
ID='ref1'>Heart Attack</concept> in …</text>…
<code code='22298006'
displayName='myocardial infarction'
        codeSystem='2.16.840.1.113883.6.96'
        codeSystemName='SNOMED CT'>
    <originalText>
<reference value='#ref1'/>
</originalText>
</code>
```

4. What is the significant difference between the Coded Ordinal (CO) and the Concept Descriptor (CD) data type (why would you use a CO instead of a CD)?

Research Questions

1. What code system uses the OID 2.16.840.1.113883.6.1? How about 2.16.840.1.113883. 6.103?
2. What is the OID for SNOMED CT? ICD-9? ICD-9-CM? RxNORM?
3. What coding systems support post-coordination?

Dates and Times

10

HL7 Version 3 allows you to say "every Tuesday for 10 minutes before 10:00 am, and Thursday 10 minutes before 2:00 pm between Labor Day and Memorial Day with the exception of holidays" as a structured set of dates. This by the way, is a dosing regimen for a treatment I used swimmers ear when swimming lessons ended at 10 am Tuesday and 2 pm Thursday during the summer months in the US. Very likely, this is a good deal more advanced that you or your application are capable of supporting.

This book will NOT get that detailed. However, it will provide the most commonly used time expressions used in CDA™ implementations.

10.1
TS Time Stamp

A time stamp is an instant in time. Since this is implicitly a quantity of time since some arbitrarily chosen epoch of time, it is part of the quantity hierarchy. The HL7 standard does not define an epoch date to be used since a system can use any epoch value and still process time stamps correctly.

The representation of the HL7 time stamp data type is based upon the ISO 8601 standard for representations of time. This is the same standard that is used in other standards for the representation of time. The ISO 8601 standard allows for punctuation characters separating portions of the time stamp to be present or absent. The HL7 use of this data type does not use punctuation characters unlike standards such as the W3C Schema Data Types. An example of the time stamp data type is shown in the figure below.

```
<effectiveTime value='20091212172151.035-0500'/>
```

Fig. 10.1 Example time stamp

This example records the date and time the example itself was produced: December 12th, 2009 at 5:21:51 and 35 ms in the afternoon in a time zone 5 h before GMT. The time stamp data type records time in the `value` XML attribute of elements that are usually named `<time>` or `<effectiveTime>` in CDA documents.

K.W. Boone, *The CDA™ Book*,
DOI: 10.1007/978-0-85729-336-7_10, © Springer-Verlag London Limited 2011

The time stamp data type is defined in the datatypes-base.xsd schema definition that is part of the CDA Release 2.0 normative edition. That schema defines the value of the time stamp using the regular expression shown below:

```
[0-9]{1,8}  |  (  [0-9]{9,14}  |  [0-9]{14,14}\.[0-9]+ )
([+\-][0-9]{1,4})?
```

Fig. 10.2 Regular expression for time stamps

This regular expression allows for the digits 0 though 9 from 1–14 times, or the 14 digits of date and time followed by a fractional number of seconds in any number of digits. When more than eight digits of a date time are present, it may be followed by an optional string beginning with either the + or − sign, followed by 1–4 digits from 0 to 9. The regular expression found in the HL7 data types schema does not prohibit illegal dates such as February 29, 2002. Furthermore, it does not restrict expressions to those containing legal values for hours, minutes or seconds. However, time stamp values which contain values outside the legal ranges are still not legal. The time stamp data type will be familiar to those who have used the HL7 Version 2 standard.

The representation of time uses two digits each to represent the century, year within century, month, day, hour, minute and second. The second can be followed by a decimal point and fractional parts of a second. Finally, the time may include a + or − sign followed by up to four digits representing the offset in hours and minutes from Universal Coordinated Time (UTC). Time stamps are restricted to legal combinations of time stamp parts.

Table 10.1 Parts of a time stamp

YYYYMMDDhhmmss.SSS±ZZzz	
YYYY	The year of the event
MM	The month in the full year
DD	The day in the month and year
hh	The hour in the day
mm	The minute in the hour
ss	The second in the minute
.SSSS	Fraction of a second
±	Direction of offset from UTC
ZZ	Hours offset from UTC
zz	Minutes offset from UTC

Synchronizing the System Clock

Systems and applications creating time stamps used in healthcare (or for any other purpose) should synchronize the time that they use with an external reference clock. Internet RFC 1305 defines a protocol known as the Network Time Protocol (NTP) that can be used to synchronize clocks over the Internet. NTP has a little brother known as the Simple Network Time Protocol (SNTP) that can also be used for this purpose. Implementations of NTP and SNTP exist for just about every operating system or platform. One or the other of these protocols is directly supported by all common operating systems.

Integrating the Healthcare Enterprise (IHE) has defined an integration profile known as Consistent Time (CT) that ensures that systems using time stamps are synchronized with a reference clock. Details of can be obtained in the IT Infrastructure Technical Framework Volumes I and II. These publications can be found on the web at http://www.ihe.net/Technical_Framework/index.cfm#IT

You can synchronize your clock on a Windows system with an external reference time server by entering the following command at a command prompt:

```
net time/setsntp:hostname
```

Simply replace `hostname` with the name of the time server. You can also configure the time server on these systems through the control panel application controlling time properties.

On the MacIntosh you can configure the time server through a Systems Preferences panel.

In UNIX environments, you need to ensure that the `ntpd` daemon is running and appropriately configured. This typically requires that the following line be included in the /etc/ntpd.conf file is included.

```
server hostname
```

The NTP protocol will slowly synchronize your clock by adjusting its slew rate, but SNTP will make large adjustments. To immediately synchronize your clock, turn off the NTP service, set your clock back 5 min and start it again.

Precision

The precision of a time stamp in a CDA document is determined by the number of digits that are provided. A time stamp can use as many digits as needed to record the time within the precision that is known. A 3 digit time stamp would be precise to the decade, a 4 digit time stamp to the year, all the way up to 14 digits to record the second within a particular date. In practice, implementations usually provide all of the digits necessary to record each part of the time stamp given. A single digit month or hour is rarely seen. However, it is perfectly legal to record only a portion of one of the parts of the time stamp.

Fractional portions of a second can record even finer degrees of precision. According to the Abstract Datatypes specification there is no theoretical limit on the number of digits allowed to record the fractional portion of the second. According to the XML ITS [§ITS 2.32] "*... the syntax is 'YYYYMMDDHHMMSS.UUUU[+|–ZZzz]' where digits can be omitted from the right side to express less precision.*" However, it is not clear whether this is meant to be a fixed limit on the number of digits because the XML Schema for data types does not limit the precision of the fractional portion.

There are also practical limits to what can be exchanged. Native data types in the Java programming language support a precision of time up to the millisecond or nanosecond (depending on the Java data types used). Data structures in C# support time precisions of up to 100 ns. In practice, time values more precise than to the second are not of much use except for detailed analysis of clinical wave forms such as those used in EKGs or EEGs. Operating system limitations restrict the precision of time stamps to be on the order of nanoseconds.

Precision is not the same as accuracy. You can record a very precise value in a time stamp. However, if the clock you are using is not accurate, the extra precision will not be of much use. Typically operating system clocks are also limited in accuracy, often having clocks that are only accurate to within a second of a specified time reference source, so more precise time values are typically only meaningful within a single system. The clocks in some of the very first personal computers were precise to about one part in 1,500,000 (about 1/18th of a second) but were much less accurate than that. I can recall one personal computer whose clock lost about 6 seconds a day (about one part in 15,000).

The value 20020229 is not a legal time stamp since February 29 is not a valid date in the year 2002. Similarly the value 200202282561 is not legal because there is neither a 25th hour nor a 61st minute in the day. However, about every 18 months leap second is introduced into UTC by an international body. The International Earth Rotation and Reference Service (IERS) is responsible for maintaining global time and reference standards. It determines when leap seconds are necessary. This is done to keep measurements of time synchronized with the earth's rotation around the sun. This means than a minute can occasionally have 61 or 62 s depending on how much adjustment is necessary. Systems which are synchronized with external reference clocks can report leap seconds in time stamps.

Time Zone

Time is usually measured according to the time in the current location, or local time. Time stamps without a time zone included are always assumed to times in a local time. Times can also be measured based on the offset from Universal Coordinated Time (otherwise known as Greenwich Mean Time). When measured in this fashion, the time zone offset in hours or hours and minutes from UTC is provided after an initial plus or minus sign. The plus or minus sign indicates that the time is ahead of or equal to UTC, or behind UTC.

In theory, the offset of UTC must always be represented using + followed by one to four zeros, but in practice the values +0, –0, +00, –00, +000, –000, +0000 and –0000 should all be recognized as a time zone that is the same as UTC.

Time zones are determined by the laws and regulations applicable in a specific location. There are time zones that are as many as 14 h ahead of or 12 h behind UTC (The HL7 Data Types standard incorrectly reports the this to be +/–12 h). Some regions have used time zones that are 20, 25 or even 43 min and 8 s different from UTC but today the offsets are more typically based on hours, with the occasional half or quarter hour.

The impact of time zone on a time stamp can be as much as 26 h, or slightly more than a single day. Therefore HL7 prohibits the use of time zones on time stamps where the precision does not include the hour of the day. This is because the variation introduced by the time zone is less than the precision of the result.

Time zones are typically not used in time stamps where the date has some administrative or legal significance. For example, a person's date of birth does not usually include a time zone since conversion to another time zone could incorrectly alter the date of birth. However, it may be relevant when this time is of clinical significance (e.g., for treatment of a newborn).

10.2
IVL_TS Interval of Time

The interval of time data type is often used to record a time interval over which some observation or event occurred or is intended to occur. Intervals of time are be specified using at most any two of the following components. Since a Time stamp is a physical quantity, the IVL_TS type in the CDA schema follows the same rules for other intervals described on page 44.

Note that comparing intervals with timestamps to determine whether the timestamp is in the interval may generate unexpected results. Can 6:00 am on January 27th, 2010 be found in the interval from January 20th, 2010 to January 27th, 2010. Before you answer that question, answer this one: Is 7.25 in the interval between 0 and 7? Of course it is not. These two questions are identical; let us see how that works.

As previously mentioned, date arithmetic can be performed using any arbitrary date as the beginning of the epoch. So, we now treat January 20th, 2010 as the epoch date. The lower and upper boundary dates of the interval can be represented as a physical quantity using days as the measurement unit. The first date is represented 0 days from the epoch date, and the second is 7 days from the epoch date. Computing the representation for 6:00 am on January 27th, 2010 generates 7.25.

While the result may be unexpected, it is not inaccurate.

The confusion results from the fact that timestamps can also be promoted to intervals based on the precision in which they are provided. The timestamp for January 27th, 2010, when promoted to an interval, includes the entire day of that date, but interval boundaries are not promoted to an interval when being used.

10.3
PIVL_TS Periodic Interval of Time

The Periodic Interval of Time data type is used to record repeating periodic events. You can think of this data type as a representation of a pulse waveform.

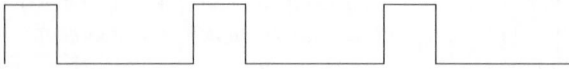

In order to fully represent the pulse, you need to know the width of the period (or its inverse, which is the frequency), the width of the pulse and the phase of the waveform. Sometimes the pulse width is effectively 0, just marking the start of different events, as shown below. Often the exact phase will not be known.

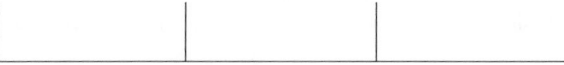

Medications are often administered on a daily basis, several times a day (e.g., three times a day). The PIVL_TS data type allows the period between these events to be recorded. Some treatments are required to occur for a specific period of time at a given frequency (e.g., PT for 1 h three times a week)

As shown in the examples, physicians often communicate regimens using the frequency rather than the period, but in the HL7 Data Types Release 1.0, you express the period rather than the frequency. The institutionSpecified XML attribute provides a mechanism to indicate which representation better reflects the intent.

<period> (See PQ Physical Quantity on Page 41)

The <period> XML element specifies the amount of time that elapses between events. The unit XML attribute indicates the time unit and is typically measured in hours, minutes, seconds or days, depending on the purpose for the periodic interval (see Table 10.2 below).

Table 10.2 Common time units

Unit code	Description
s	Second
min	Minute
h	Hour
d	Day
wk	Week
mo	Month

This XML attribute must be present in any reasonable implementation to indicate the units of time. The `value` XML attribute indicates the number of time units that occur between each period. It must be expressed as a real number.

institutionSpecified (See BL Boolean on Page 39)

The `institutionSpecified` XML attribute differentiates between period specifications (e.g., every 8 h) and frequency specifications (e.g., three times per day) that would otherwise have identical representations. Even though the average frequency is the same for these two, the difference between them could have a serious impact on patient care. When the period between events is critical, this XML attribute must have a value of `false`. When the time between events can be adjusted by the organization or person responsible for the event to fit other activities; the XML attribute may have a value of `true`. If this attribute is not specified, implementations must act as if the value is `false` (this is the default value).

\<phase\> (See TS Timestamp on Page 95)

If the PIVL_TS is a pulse waveform, more than just the period of the waveform to fully represent it. The starting point and length of the pulse are also needed.

This information is represented in the `<phase>` XML element. This element gives the starting time and length for the pulse. Because it uses the IVL_TS data type, it can be represented in as many as eight different ways. I recommend representing it using the `<low>` and `<width>` XML elements. These most closely represent the concepts of starting time and length of the pulse. If the event does not really have a specified duration (e.g., just marks the administration of a medication), you need not specify the width of the pulse. If the amount of time is important, but the starting time is not relevant, it can be omitted and just the `<width>` can be specified (e.g., 1 h of physical therapy three times per week, or brush your teeth three times a day for 1 min).

The `<phase>` element is often absent in many uses of PIVL_TS because it is either not known, or not relevant. The starting time found in the `<low>` element of phase need not be the actual starting time of the first event. It can be any starting time that is synchronized with the frequency of the event. Note that when `institutionSpecified` is `true`, the starting time of phase can effectively be ignored (since the institution may use a different starting time), and only the `<width>` is important.

10.4
EIVL_TS Event-Related Periodic Interval of Time

The event related periodic interval of time is used to represent periodic events that are tied to meals and sleeping.

<event> (See CS Coded Simple on Page 91)

The <event> element contains the specific periodic event that the activity is related to in the code XML attribute. The codes are fixed to those found in Table 10.3.

<offset> (See IVL_* Numeric Intervals on Page 44)

If the activity being reported or scheduled occurs at the time of the event then no <offset> XML element is needed. However, if the event is to occur before or after the event, or the activity has duration, then you need to specify the offset and duration using the IVL_PQ data type.

This works similarly to the way that the <phase> element is used in the PIVL_TS data type. In the EIVL_TS data type, the start of the interval is specified as an offset in time units from the event. *This offset is in the direction specified by the code. The Offset column in Table 10.3 indicates whether the direction for <offset> is forwards (F) in time, backwards (B) in time, or not used with that event (X). To avoid duplicate representations offsets should only be positive values.* In Data Types Release 2.0, which will be used with CDA Release 3.0, the definition of offset is changed to elimination the need for code specific interpretation. The end result will be cleaner.

Table 10.3 Event related timing codes

Code	Offset	Description
AC	B	Before meal (from lat. ante cibus)
ACM	B	Before breakfast (from lat. ante cibus matutinus)
ACT	B	Before lunch (from lat. ante cibus diurnus)
ACV	B	Before dinner (from lat. ante cibus vespertinus)
HS	X[a]	The hour of sleep
IC	X	Between meals (from lat. inter cibus)
ICD	X	Between lunch and dinner
ICM	X	Between breakfast and lunch
ICV	X	Between dinner and the hour of sleep
PC	F	After meal (from lat. post cibus)
PCD	F	After lunch (from lat. post cibus diurnus)
PCM	F	After breakfast (from lat. post cibus matutinus)
PCV	F	After dinner (from lat. post cibus vespertinus)

Contents of this table are drawn from the HL7 Vocabulary Standard with permission

[a]The hour of sleep does not have any implied direction. Would it make more sense to schedule something before or after the hour of sleep? What is the normal direction of time? The common answers to these questions are competing reasons for using either direction, and so my recommendation is to avoid the problem by not using <offset> with that event

The offset appears in the `value` XML attribute. The time units appear in the unit XML attribute. See Table 10.2 above for UCUM codes for common time units.

10.5
GTS Generic Timing Specification

The Generic Timing Specification allows complex timings to be expressed as a set of time intervals using a variety of different set operations, including intersections, unions, differences, and a complex operation known as a periodic hull. The periodic hull operation essentially allows pairs of operands in two different sets to be used as the boundaries for intervals between them. This allows:

- A set expression to be constructed to generate all of the dates for the US Memorial day holiday (the last Monday in May).
- Another set expression to be constructed to generate all of the dates for the US Labor day holiday (the first Monday in September).
- A third set expression to be constructed containing all of the intervals between the items in these two sets (all the "summer vacation days" commonly taken off by students in the school year).

Almost any schedule imaginable can be represented in this way, including many of effectively infinite length.

10.6
Use of Time Data Types with Medications

The most complex use of the time data types described above in the CDA standard appears when describing the frequency of medication administration. The `<substanceAdministration>` XML element specifies dose frequency in `<effectiveTime>` elements using the GTS data type. That means that you have to build up the complete expression using a combination of the types described above.

There are many ways in which this can be legally accomplished using the HL7 time data types, and information systems that are based on the HL7 RIM will treat each of them as identical. However, the reality is that systems rarely deal with administration timings at this level of complexity. Integrating the Healthcare Enterprise established the convention that timings would be encoded using one of the following two representations:

- A single time stamp representing the time of a single administration event.
- An interval expressing the start and stop times of the dosing regimen, intersected with the dose frequency, expressed either as a periodic interval of time (PIVL_TS) or as an event related periodic interval of time (EIVL_TS).

If more complex than what could be handled by the above, the regimen would merely need to be expressed in the human readable text.

The example in the figure below shows a single administration on a given date.

```
<effectiveTime xsi:type='TS' value='200509010118'/>
```

Fig. 10.3 Once on a given date

The next four examples show a five day regimen at various frequencies using the PIVL_TS data type.

```
<effectiveTime xsi:type='IVL_TS'>
   <low value='20100708'/><high value='20100712'/>
</effectiveTime>
<effectiveTime xsi:type='PIVL_TS'
 institutionSpecified='true' operator='A'>
   <period value='12' unit='h' />
</effectiveTime>
```

Fig. 10.4 Twice a day (BID)

```
<effectiveTime xsi:type='IVL_TS'>
   <low value='20100708'/><high value='20100712'/>
</effectiveTime>
<effectiveTime xsi:type='PIVL_TS'
 institutionSpecified='false' operator='A'>
   <period value='12' unit='h' />
</effectiveTime>
```

Fig. 10.5 Every 12 h (Q12H)

```
<effectiveTime xsi:type='IVL_TS'>
   <low value='20100708'/><high value='20100712'/>
</effectiveTime>
<effectiveTime xsi:type='PIVL_TS'
 institutionSpecified='true' operator='A'>
   <period value='8' unit='h' />
</effectiveTime>
```

Fig. 10.6 Three times a day (TID)

```
<effectiveTime xsi:type='IVL_TS'>
   <low value='20100708'/><high value='20100712'/>
</effectiveTime>
<effectiveTime xsi:type='PIVL_TS'
 institutionSpecified='false' operator='A'>
   <period value='8' unit='h' />
</effectiveTime>
```

Fig. 10.7 Every 8 h (Q8H)

The following example shows two different five day regimens using the EIVL_TS data type.

```
<effectiveTime xsi:type='IVL_TS'>
   <low value='20100708'/><high value='20100712'/>
</effectiveTime>
<effectiveTime xsi:type='EIVL' operator='A'>
   <event code='ACM'/>
</effectiveTime>
```

Fig. 10.8 Before breakfast

```
<effectiveTime xsi:type='EIVL' operator='A'>
   <event code='ACM'/>
   <offset>
       <width value='10' unit='min'/>
   </offset>
</effectiveTime>
```

Fig. 10.9 Before breakfast for 10 min

Summary

- Timestamps appear in the form YYYYMMDDhhmmss.SSS±ZZzz where each letter is a digit
- Components of the time stamp are ordered from most to least significant.
- The length of the timestamp determines its precision.
- The IVL_TS data type looks like other intervals in HL7 Version 3 Data types.
- Comparing intervals requires care because the precision of interval boundaries is not considered in comparisons.
- The PIVL_TS data type allows one to specify a "pulse-like" waveform.

- The institutionSpecified component of the periodic interval (PIVL_TS) affects how it is interpreted in important ways.
- Event based Intervals can be specified based on sleeping and eating periods using the EIVL_TS data type.

Questions

1. How would you represent your birth date in a time stamp? Would it contain a time zone? Why or why not?
2. Is 20081231185960-0500 a legal time stamp value? Why or why not?
3. What does the presence of the institutionSpecified attribute do to a periodic interval?
4. Which of the following is the best representation of the interval covering the entire day of January 20, 1965?

```
<time value='19650120'/>
<time>
    <low   value='196501200000'/>
    <high value='196501201259'/>
</time>
<time>
    <low   value='19650120'/>
    <high value='19650121'/>
</time>
```

5. How would you express 1 h before bedtime? What are the problems with this representation?

Research Questions

1. How would you represent a variable time interval such as every 4–6 h? What policy issues does this raise?
2. What is the appropriate XML representation for the regimen of 5 min every Tuesday at 1 pm and every Thursday at 10 am between Memorial Day and Labor Day?
3. There is an even more accurate way to describe the entire day of January 20, 1965 that is not listed in question 4 above. It uses an attribute not described in this book. What is it?

Collections

11

The HL7 Abstract Data Types specification includes several types of abstract collections of different data types, including bags, sets and lists. These collection data types can be used with any of the other simpler data types. Unlike other object models, the HL7 collection types do not derive sets or lists from the bag collection type, even though a set and a list could be thought of as specializations of the bag type.

Few of these collection types are used directly by CDA™ (the most commonly used is the Set collection type). The Message Element type column of the CDA Hierarchical Descriptor is a good place to look for this information. All data types defined in the CDA schemas, including the various collection types can appear in the `<value>` element of the `<observation>` element. One must simply use the appropriate `xsi:type` declaration to use these types.

Most implementations of CDA can be understood without delving into the details of the collection data types.

The collection data types in CDA work only with quantities (including time stamps) and coded concepts. They do not work with the multimedia, text or demographics data types.

One of the more difficult things about using the collection data types is determining which type to use in the CDA schemas to represent a collection component. This is because the datatypes.xsd schema defines only those data types necessary to represent the various collection types, without creating types for more constrained uses. For example, an interval of PQ can represent a single physical quantity as well as a range of quantities. So, there is a type defined in the schema that supports a bag of intervals of PQ (BXIT_IVL_PQ), but there is no type defined that supports just a bag of PQ. If you want to represent something using a bag of physical quantities, you need to use the BXIT_IVL_PQ type.

11.1
BAG Bag

A bag is an unordered collection of items that may be duplicated. In the XML, a bag of any data type is usually written as a sequence of items using the data type associated with the bag. The order does not matter, so this information can be written back out in a different order without any change in the meaning. The CDA standard does not use the BAG data type directly.

K.W. Boone, *The CDA™ Book*,
DOI: 10.1007/978-0-85729-336-7_11, © Springer-Verlag London Limited 2011

Bags of codes can be used in <value> elements using the BXIT_CD data type. Since all coded data types derive from CD, you can use this type to create bags of simpler coded types.

Bags of physical quantities, integers or real numbers should use the BXIT_IVL_PQ type in the datatypes.xsd schema. This works because IVL_PQ can also be used to represent a PQ, and PQ is sufficient to represent a real or integer. This type is sufficient to represent the information but will not constrain an implementation to the use of PQ, INT or REAL representations via the schema. Those constraints must be applied using other technologies.

11.2
SET Set

A set is an unordered collection of unique items where each item may not be repeated. In a CDA XML instance, a set of any data type is usually written as a sequence of items using the data type associated with the set. Like the bag, the order of items in the set does not matter, so the information can be written back out in a different order without any change in the meaning.

In CDA Release 2.0, the Set type is used with addresses, names, identifiers, telecommunications addresses, and most participations and act relationships, but these are anonymous types in the schema. An anonymous type is one which is locally defined in a schema in a way that does not allow it to be reused elsewhere. But that does not prevent you from including a set of these data types in the CDA instance because some data elements like the <value> element in an <observation> allow use of ANY. You would just repeat the <value> element as many times as you like and use the set member type (e.g., ADDR, PN, II, TEL, et cetera).

The set collection type can also be used with a continuous range (e.g., real numbers or physical quantities). The most common use of this capability in CDA is found where the General Timing Specification (GTS) appears. GTS is simply a SET of Time Stamps.

Sets can be created by various set operations, including union, difference and intersection with another set. The various SXCM types defined in the datatypes.xsd schema of the CDA standard are used to create sets of codes, integers, real numbers, time stamps or physical quantities.

Operator

The SXCM types in the schema include an operator XML attribute which indicates how the new item impacts the set that was constructed thus far. Table 11.1 below describes the possible operations.

The default value of the operator XML attribute is I, which means that the item will be included in the new set.

Table 11.1 Set operations

Operator	Name	Description
A	Intersect	Produce a new set by taking the intersection of the set generated thus far with the set that uses this operator.
E	Exclude	Remove the set using this operator from the set that was generated thus far.
H	Convex hull	Form a new set by creating the smallest range containing both the set using this operator and the set generated thus far. For example, if set A contains the number 1, and set B contains the number 5, then the convex hull of A and B contains the numbers from 1 to 5 inclusive.
I	Include	Add this set to the set generated thus far (the set union operation).
P	Periodic hull	Generate a new set that consists of the convex hull generated from the pairs of corresponding members of each set.

Contents of this table are drawn from the HL7 Vocabulary Standard with permission. Columns 1 and 2 come directly from the standard. Column 3 is the author's interpretation

11.3
IVL Interval

The interval is a range from one point to another, and so is another type of set. Intervals can only be with HL7 data types that represent quantities and are described in more detail under the Quantity Data type on page 39.

11.4
LIST List

A list is an ordered collection of items that may be duplicated. In the XML, a list of any data type is written as a sequence of items using the data type associated with the list in the appropriate order. Since the order matters, this information must be written back out in the same order as the original to avoid any change in meaning. In CDA, the List collection type only appears in the `<value>` element found in the `<regionOfInterest>` element. These values are used to specify coordinates on an image.

However, LIST can also be used as the data type for `<value>` in an `<observation>` element.

HL7 defines two additional List data types; a generated list (GLIST) and a sampled list (SLIST). The GLIST data type generates a list algorithmically, much like the "FOR" statement found in many programming languages. The Sampled List allows data from a sampling device (e.g., an analog to digital signal converter connected to some input signal) to be transmitted using raw output.

Summary

- Sets, lists and bags are all different types of collections that can be used with many HL7 data types.
- Sets do not allow duplication and can specify continuous or discontinuous ranges.
- The interval data type allows for the creation of a continuous range and is also a set.
- Sets can be created by using a variety of different set operations.
- Lists are ordered and can allow duplicated content.
- Bags are unordered and can allow duplicated content.

Questions

1. What are the most commonly used collection data types in CDA Release 2.0?
2. Where can you easily find the information needed to answer the question above?

Research Questions

1. What schema type from datatypes.xsd would you use to represent a bag, set and list of codes respectively?
2. What schema type from datatypes.xsd would you use to represent a bag a bag of integers or real numbers?
3. Why is there no GTS data type defined in datatypes.xsd? What schema type would you use instead?
4. What is a periodic hull and why is it important?

HL7 Version 3 Modeling
12

The HL7 Reference Information Model (or RIM for short) is the UML model for health-care information from which the CDA™ Standard is derived. A simplified diagram of the RIM appears in the figure below (the smaller classes are not used in CDA). This diagram shows that the RIM has six base classes from which all other HL7 classes are derived. *These six base classes are known as the backbone of the RIM.*

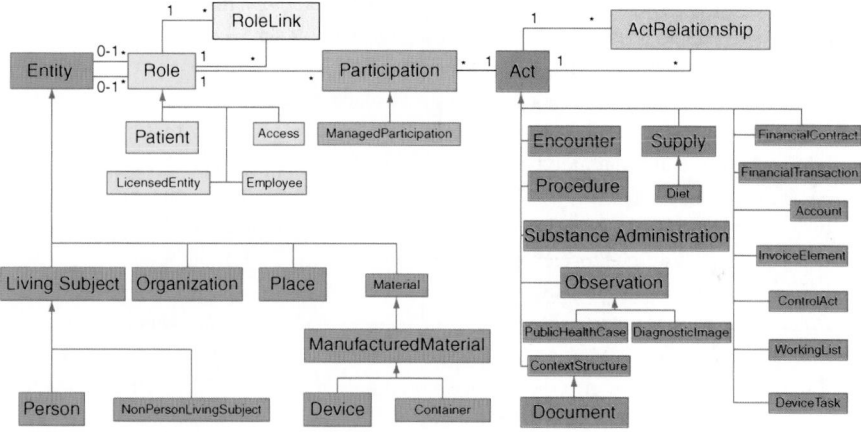

Fig. 12.1 The HL7 RIM

Learning to work with these classes in critical for understanding how HL7 Version 3 works.

12.1
The RIM Backbone Classes

The six base classes of the RIM can be connected a very small number of controlled ways, providing a basic syntax for the creation sentences or *clinical statements*. The six base classes are effectively the *parts of speech* of the HL7 RIM. Learning to speak in these six

K.W. Boone, *The CDA™ Book*,
DOI: 10.1007/978-0-85729-336-7_12, © Springer-Verlag London Limited 2011

basic classes becomes the challenge of any HIT developer who wants to use HL7 Version 3 specifications, including the CDA.

Act

Acts are the verbs in the RIM. They represent various actions that can be taken in a clinical statement. Like German, the Act is the crux of the sentence, but unlike German, the "verb" comes first in most human interactions with the RIM. There are 20 different types of verbs (act classes) defined in the RIM, of which 7 appear in CDA: Act, Document, Observation, PatientEncounter, Procedure, SubstanceAdministration and Supply.

Mood

Like verbs in other languages, the verbs in HL7 Version 3 have an attribute known as *mood*, although in most cases most people would recognize this as *tense*, since the most common uses have more to do with time than *mood*. The HL7 moods fall into two general categories: the "completion track", and "predicates". The moods in the *completion track* represent various transitions of an Act from definition to intent to completed event. The transition from definition to intent to event in the RIM is exemplified by comparing it to the transitions from a clinical guideline (a definition for care) to a care plan (the care intended to be performed) and finally to the care that has been provided (the actual care events).

DEF – Acts in definition mood define a template for what is or should occur or appear. These are definitional statements.

INT – Acts in Intent mood (of which there are several sub-varieties, including RQO for request or order) describe those events that are intended to occur in the future.

EVN – Acts in event mood describe what has occurred.

Predicate moods describe criteria, goals or options. These are more nebulous future or possible kinds of acts.

EVN.CRT – The event criteria mood is commonly used in CDA to identify acts that specify a precondition for certain acts (e.g., PRN for pain is a precondition).

GOL – Acts in the goal mood describes an expectation or hope to make an observation with a desired value in the future.

ActRelationship

ActRelationships link acts together to form more complex sentences. They are the conjunctions of the HL7 language. Unfortunately, HL7 seems to have developed conjunctivitis, because there are an inflaming number of ways that acts can be joined together.

Participation

Participations are the *subjects* and *objects* of the clinical statements made up in RIM sentences. Each act can have zero or more participants. Each participant in the act has one or more roles. The participant class links an Act to a Role.

Role

A role describes a relationship between two entities, for example, a patient and the specimen extracted from them, or a physician and the organizational context in which they provide care. These two entities are known as the *player* and the *scoper*. The Player takes part in a role within the context of the scoping entity. The RIM defines five different kinds of role, the base Role class (which is the only one use by CDA), and four specializations (Employee, Patient, LicensedEntity and Access). The specializations of Role are not used by CDA because the additional features they support are simply not needed by it.

Roles and Participations

The ISO Privilege Management and Access Control standard describes two different types of roles for an entity, called structural and functional roles. A *structural role* describes the role of an entity that is based on its qualities, or what it IS. A *functional role* describes the role of an entity that is based on its relationship with other entities, or on what it DOES. Structural roles are static, functional roles are more dynamic, and often more contextual. The attending physician for one patient on a ward may not be the attending physician for all patients, but is still a physician.

To give an example in healthcare: A person in the role of physician is in that role by virtue of their education and licensure. This is a structural role. That same person would be in the functional role of attending or consulting physician by virtue of their relationship with the patient, and the fact that they are authorized (perhaps by their education and licensure) to be in that role.

To simplify, assume that there is a function of baby deliverer. Most commonly the person playing this function would be an obstetrician. However, that functional role could also be played by an ambulance attendant, a policeman, or simply the spouse of the expectant mother. The functional role that is being performed is delivering the baby, and it need NOT be played by someone qualified by their structural role. A common scenario in Television drama occurs when a passenger lands a plan. The functional role is "plane lander", and while the ideal case would include someone qualified to perform this role, like a pilot, it could be handled by another person in an emergency.

The Role class in HL7 describes a structural role. The Participation class describes a functional role. Roles and participations can be applied to more than just people. A medication can be in the functional role of being a blood thinner (what it does), and have the structural role of being aspirin (what it is).

Entity

Entities are the formal nouns of HL7. These are the persons, places or things associated with providing healthcare. There are ten different kinds of entities in the RIM, six of which are used in CDA (Person, Place, Organization, Device, Entity and ManufacturedMaterial).

RoleLink

The RoleLink is a very rare animal indeed in V3 Modeling, and is not seen at all in CDA. This class describes the relationships between two roles (e.g., the supervisor of a provider, the operator of a modality, the attending provider assigned to a patient).

12.2
HL7 Modeling and UML

HL7 uses its own representation of UML to reflect the use of these six backbone classes. Each class has its own color and shape to represent the stereotypes of Act, ActRelationship, Participation, Role, Entity and RoleLink, and they only connect in certain ways. An Act can have ActRelationships and Participations attached. Participations point to Roles, and Roles point to Entities.

The ActRelationship, Participation and RoleLink classes are UML association classes. In UML, an *association class* describes the relationship between two classes in more detail. The Role class can also be viewed as an imperfect association class. In UML the two ends of the relationship must always be present, but in HL7 Version 3, the scoper and player Entity classes that are associated with each other through the Role class need not always appear.

The figure above shows the HL7 and UML representations of the six core classes as they relate to each other. HL7 representations use square boxes for Acts, Roles and Entities

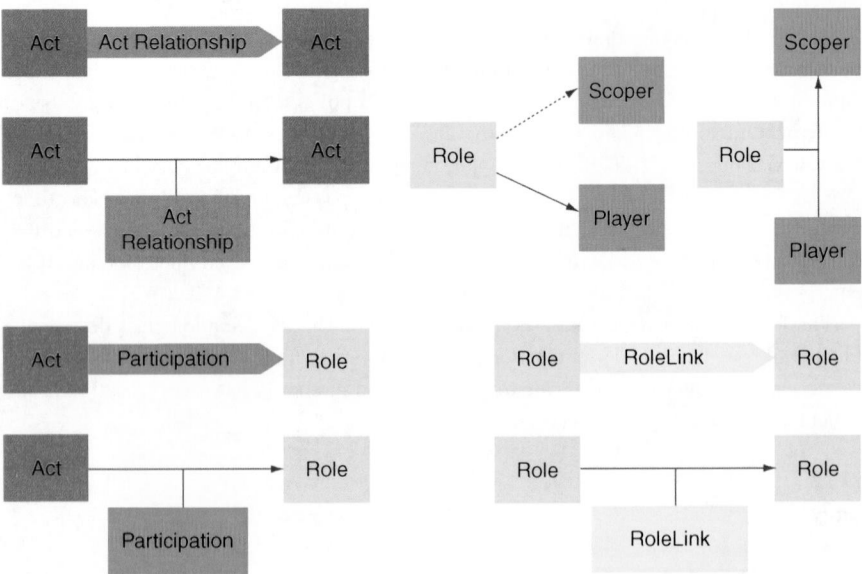

Fig. 12.2 The RIM secret decoder ring

(Scoper and Player), and arrow shaped boxes for ActRelationship, Participation, and RoleLink. UML representations for these use square boxes for all classes and T-shaped lines connecting all the components. The HL7 notation is a little bit more compact in diagramming, but confusing for those who have never seen it before.

HL7 Version 3 modeling has a few other digressions from UML modeling. Only classes are described in Version 3, never interfaces. Classes have class attributes, but no methods. In part this is because most HL7 models describe information being sent in a message (a method call) to an interface.

Finally, there is the rather common choice box found in HL7 Version 3 that is effectively a union of different RIM classes.

Hungarian Notation

HL7 used a naming convention similar to the Hungarian notation [1] used in some programming languages when it named the various RIM attributes. The final word at the end of the name of the class attribute almost always tells you the data type associated with it. This makes it fairly easy for humans to understand each of the class attributes represented in the XML. This convention is a general principal applied to HL7 class attribute names, but there are a few exceptions. Table 12.1 below lists the words or abbreviations and the data types associated with each. HL7 class attributes appear in the XML in what is called camel case (So called because the words have humps in the middle due to the mixed capitalization). Names that would normally contain spaces for human readability are not allowed in XML. To make these names easier for people to read, HL7 capitalizes the first letter of each separate word in the name.

Table 12.1 HL7 class attribute naming convention

Suffix	Data type	HL7 data types
Addr	Address	AD
Code	Concept descriptor	CD, CE, CO or CS
Desc	Description	ED
Expr	Expression	ST
Id	Identifier	II
Ind[a]	Boolean	BL, BN
Name	Entity name	EN, PN, ON
Number	Integer	INT
Quantity	Quantity	PQ, REAL
Telecom	Telecommunications address	TEL
Text	Text	ED, ST
Time	Time and date	TS, GTS

[a]Ind is short for Indicator

Reading an HL7 Diagram

HL7 diagrams are simply a variant of UML as described above. Each figure (box or arrow shape) contains the class name and then the class attributes and their properties.

Properties of Class Attributes

Class attributes appear in each class in using a HL7 short-hand notation. The first component is the class attribute name. The figure below shows the class attributes of the author association class.

---

functionCode: CE CWE [0..1] <= *ParticipationFunction*

contextControlCode*: CS CNE [1..1] <= " *OP* "

time*: TS [1..1]

Fig. 12.3 Class attributes in HL7 diagrams

HL7 has specific terms it uses to describe conformance to a model. Class attributes are optional, required or mandatory. An *optional* class attribute is just that, it can be included or not, and if included, it may contain a flavor of null (be empty). A *required* class attribute must always be included, but can contain a flavor of null. Finally, a *mandatory* class attribute must always be included and cannot contain a flavor of null. Required class attributes are followed by an asterisk, and mandatory class attributes appear in bold and are followed by an asterisk. In the example shown above, functionCode is optional, contextControlCode is mandatory, and time is required.

The next part of the class attribute identifies the data type. For the example above: The functionCode class attribute use the CE data type (Coded with Equivalents). The contextControlCode class attribute uses the CS data type (Coded Simple). The time class attribute uses the TS data type (Time stamp). The number of times the data element is permitted to appear (its cardinality) shows up in between brackets. Items which are either *required* or *mandatory* will always have a lower bound of 1. If there is a default value for the attribute, it will appear in between quotes.

When class attributes use the CD data type (Concept Descriptor), or any data type derived from it (e.g., CE or CS as shown above), there are two other pieces of information needed to describe the vocabulary allowed in the coded concept. The first of these is an indication whether that vocabulary must be used, or is simply the recommended one. The acronym CWE stands for coded with exceptions, and when appearing after the data type, indicates that the specified vocabulary is recommended. The acronym CNE stands for Coded no exceptions and indicates that the specified vocabulary must be used.

The second information component identifies the concept domain, vocabulary, value set or fixed value required by the standard. A *concept domain* is simply a named set of concepts with no associated vocabulary or value set. Vocabularies and value sets are defined in Chap. 8. Fixed values are simply selected codes from a vocabulary. Every HL7 Vocabulary has an associated Concept Domain with the same name.

But you cannot visually distinguish between HL7 Vocabularies, Concept Domains, value sets and fixed values. The following rules of thumb will help:

1. HL7 Vocabulary and Concept Domain names are expressed in camel case (e.g., CamelCase).
2. HL7 Value Set names always begin with x_
3. HL7 Codes are all sequences of uppercase letters and numbers, but
4. HL7 Codes are hierarchical, so the standard could mean: this exact code (a fixed value), or this code and anything under it (a value set).
5. In later versions of the RIM modeling tools (And therefore not found in the CDA Standard), a less than or equals sign <= before the vocabulary constraint expresses "includes this code and all descendants", and an equal sign = expresses "just this code".
6. If there is both an HL7 concept domain and an HL7 vocabulary, then the constraint indicates that the HL7 Vocabulary is being required or recommended.

After CDA Release 2.0 was completed, additional refinements were made in modeling tools that allowed the vocabulary constraints to be visually distinguished in the models.

Class Name and Structural Attributes

Fundamental features of each class appearing in the R-MIM diagram appear at the top of each class. Examples appear below.

Fig. 12.4 Interpreting the first part of a RIM class

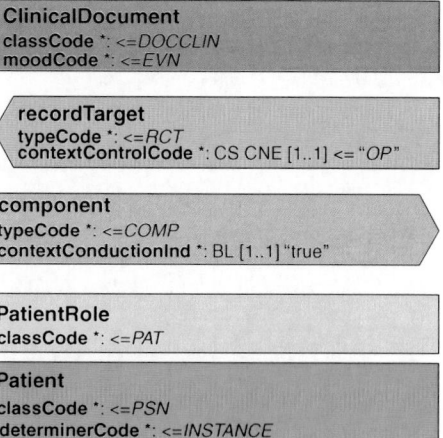

The name of the class appears at the very top of the box or arrow used to represent each class. This is the name that will be used in the XML representation inside the CDA Schema. The classes appearing above will have XML that looks like that shown the figure below.

```
<ClinicalDocument classCode='DOCCLIN' moodCode='EVN'>
   ...
</ClinicalDocument>
<component typeCode='COMP' contextConductionInd='true'>
   ...
</component>
<recordTarget typeCode='RCT' contextControlCode='OP'>
   ...
</recordTarget>
<patientRole classCode='PAT'>
   ...
</patientRole>
<patient classCode='PSN' determinerCode='INSTANCE'>
   ...
</patient>
```

Fig. 12.5 XML from the example class

Class attributes that appear following the class name in Fig. 12.4 are what are known as *structural attributes*. Structural attributes convey information related to how the RIM works, rather than specific clinical content. Structural attributes appear as XML attributes in XML representations. Table 12.2 below lists structural attributes important to CDA.

Table 12.2 Structural attributes

RIM class	Structural attribute	Purpose
Act	classCode	Identifies the RIM class used.
	moodCode	Describes the tense and mode of the act.
	negationInd	Indicates that the act itself is negated.
ActRelationship	typeCode	Describes the subtype of ActRelationship.
	inversionInd	Indicates that the direction of the relationship is inverted from the direction of serialization.
	contextConductionInd	Indicates whether context is conveyed through the relationship.
Entity	classCode	Indicates the RIM class used.
	determinerCode	Indicates whether this class describes an kind of entity or represents an instance of one.
Participation	typeCode	Describes the subtype of Participation.
	contextControlCode	Indicates how this participation changes the context.
Role	classCode	Identifies the RIM class used.

You will note that class names appearing in HL7 Models often differ from the class names used in the HL7 RIM. This is because HL7 modeling works by *restriction*. The RIM describes everything that can be said in HL7 Version 3. The document and message models further restrict the communication. The classes used in documents or messaging are restricted models of their RIM counterparts. Because of the way XML Schema works, two different elements with the same element name must have the same structure. This prevents an XML representation from being created that enforces one set of rules for an element named `<act>` in one place and another set of rules somewhere else. So, each restricted model needs a new name. HL7 invented a term for these restricted models. They are known as clones or class clones, since they are (restricted) copies of an existing RIM class. The name of the restricted class is the clone name. In HL7 Version 3, clones are not identical to their ancestor.

Class and Type Codes

The first class attribute after the class name (or the clone name to use HL7 speak) indicates which of the RIM classes or subtypes of a RIM class the clone originated from. This will be named either `classCode` or `typeCode` depending on the RIM class it originated from. RIM classes that form a hierarchy (like Act, Entity and Role) use `classCode`. The `classCode` identifies the specific RIM class being represented. The association classes do not have different forms, so these are simply subtypes of these RIM classes and use `typeCode`.

Mood

The next class attribute appearing the RIM Act class is the `moodCode`. In grammar, mood and tense are two different axes which can be used to describe the way a verb is used. In HL7 Version 3, mood and tense are conflated (as they often are in many languages) into the `moodCode`. This attribute indicates how the act is being used, and in what tense it is being described.

HL7 Version 3 has a number of different `moodCode` values. The most important ones are described in more detail in Table 12.3 below.

Table 12.3 Values of `moodCode`

Name	Code	Description
Definition	DEF	A description of an act that can occur.
Intent	INT	The intent for an act to occur in the future
Proposal	PRP	A proposal to perform an act in the future
Promise	PRMS	The promise to perform an act in the future
Request or order	RQO	A request or order to perform an act in the future
Event	EVN	The actual occurrence of an act.
Event criteria	EVN.CRT	An event that must occur or criteria that must be applicable before another event can happen
Expectation	EXPEC	The expectation that something may occur in the future
Goal	GOL	The hope, expectation or desire that something does occur in the future

The first six mood code values described above are part of what HL7 calls the *Act Completion* track. Moods in the *Act Completion* track describe various stages of care. These represent transitions from definition (e.g., a clinical guideline for care), to intent (a plan of care), to event (a sequence of care events that have taken place). Intent can be shaded into finer distinctions of proposed, promised, and ordered, each of which imply a greater degree of commitment.

The remaining moods fall into the *predicate track*. Once again, grammarians and linguists will recognize that a predicate is the component of the sentence that modifies or conditions the subject of the sentence. In CDA, Acts using the predicate moods are used to deal with preconditions and goals.

Class Attributes

Negation of an Act

When making clinical statements, it is almost as important to be able to say that something has not occurred or was not done (or shouldn't occur or be done) as it is to say that it has. The Review of Systems and Physical Examination sections of many clinical documents often contain clinical statements that report the lack of a symptom or physical finding. The *negationInd* attribute on the Act class allows the specific content of the act to be negated. Negation applies to the *descriptive properties* of the act. Acts have two kinds of properties, inert and descriptive. *Inert properties* of an act are the attributes and associations that are independent of the mood of the act (e.g., identifier or author). The descriptive properties of the act indicate the why, what, when, where, how, and in some cases, the who.

One way to distinguish between descriptive and inert properties is to ask the question of whether the property is about the act (descriptive) or the record of the act (inert). Relationships between Acts and participations in acts are also properties of acts, and can be inert or descriptive in HL7 Version 3. Fortunately, the ActRelationships used in CDA are always descriptive properties.

The following table indicates the most common inert properties found in the CDA standard.

Table 12.4 Inert properties in CDA

Source	Element name
Act attributes	moodCode
	id
	text
	statusCode
	confidentialityCode
	languageCode
Participations	author (AUT)
	authenticator (AUTHEN)
	dataEnterer (ENT)
	legalAuthenticator (LA)
	informant (INF)
	informationRecipient (IRCP)
	responsibleParty (RESP)

When an act is negated in Event mood, it indicates that the specified act did not occur. When negated in Intent moods it indicates that it should not occur. In predicate moods, it indicates that the criteria should not be present.

The more descriptive properties that are included in a negated act, the more restricted the negation is. If the act is administration of aspirin, and it is negated, this indicates that aspirin was not administered. If the act is administration of aspirin on September 3, 2010, then its negation indicates that no aspirin was administered on that date, but it could well have been administered on another date. If the act indicated aspirin given orally on September 3, 2010, then its negation is that no orally administered aspirin was given on that date, but it does not preclude any other method or date of administration.

One of the difficulties with negation occurs with the fact that code and value in observation convey somewhat different pieces of information. Consider the following two statements:

1. Evidence of a heart attack was not observed.
2. No evidence of a heart attack was observed.

The first statement indicates that no observation was performed that showed any evidence of a heart attack. It could indicate that a number of observations were performed, and none of them indicated evidence of a heart attack, or that no observations were performed at all. The second statement is more specific. It indicates that an observation was made that there is no evidence of a heart attack. The former statement is more general, the latter more specific. The question occurs as to which interpretation is meant when an observation of evidence of a heart attack is negated.

This question was significant enough to cause a change to be made in the HL7 RIM after CDA Release 2 was finalized as a standard. However, this change did not affect the CDA standard because it specified use of a specific version of the RIM prior to this change. The change will be incorporated into CDA Release 3. In the meantime, the HL7 Structured Documents Workgroup has established some guidance in the use of negation in CDA Release 2.

Context Propagation

Every act in an HL7 model has associated with it a context. That context includes the participations and other acts associated with the source act. In UML these are just different associations related to the model, but in HL7 modeling, there is an added dimension. Information asserted at one level of the model is able to *propagate* or be inherited through these associations with other acts.

Thus, every clinical statement in a CDA document has an author that need not be explicitly stated. It's simply the author of the section, or if none is found there, the author of the clinical document. Context propagation is a simplifying feature of the HL7 RIM and the Implementation Technology Specification. It allows you to specify that certain properties of an Act can be inherited from other acts that are related to it.

Context propagation works because the HL7 models need to be *serialized*, or written out in some form to be transmitted or stored. That serialization format is specified in the XML ITS specification. Context is inherited down the tree in the XML representation. This allows the XPath expression `ancestor-or-self::*[cda:author][1]/`

cda:author to be used to locate the author(s) of a clinical statement. This expression works only if these contextual features are completely re-specified when modified, and if the context can always be assumed to conduct downward through the tree. The default and usually fixed settings in CDA ensure that these requirements are met.

The one case where changes can be made to context conduction is in the contextConductionInd class attribute of the entryRelationship class. If this class attribute is set to false, then no context is conducted to the clinical statements that follow. This might be done for example when duplicating clinical information from other sources where the document context simply does not apply. The challenge this introduces for consumers of the clinical document is that they no longer have an easy way to locate components of the context.

The fixed values used in the CDA R-MIM for contextControlCode and default values used for contextConductionInd make it possible to correctly interpret context using simple XPath expressions. Relatively few CDA processors are fully aware of the ITS context conduction rules. This makes it advisable to use the default settings for contextConductionInd class attribute of the entryRelationship class used by CDA when creating an instance of a CDA document.

Entities as Instances or Descriptions

The last special attribute is the determinerCode attribute found on the Entity classes. The entity class can either describe a kind of entity, or represent a specific instance of an entity. The determinerCode is set to KIND or INSTANCE respectively. If you simply describe something, (e.g., a mark 2 vorpal hip joint) or someone (e.g., a cardiologist), use KIND. However, it you are describing a specific thing (e.g., the mark 2 vorpal hip joint with serial number 2342), or person (e.g., the cardiologist Patrick Pump with id # 222-33-4444) then you would use INSTANCE.

Changes in the RIM

Over time the HL7 RIM has changed in response to various issues that have been discovered and in response to new requirements. Because CDA Release 2 uses a fixed version of the RIM, these changes have not had any impact on it.

New moods have been added to the RIM, such as Risk (RSK), which is simple the hope, expectation or desire that something DOES NOT occur in the future. The Event Criteria (EVN.CRT) mood has been deprecated as HL7 has discovered a better way to express query criteria. The negationInd attribute has been split into two components, actionNegationInd (on Act), and valueNegationInd on observation because it was shown that negation was ambiguous in its application on the action or the value. These changes will need to be addressed during the development of CDA Release 3.0.

RIM Attributes for the Class

The remainder of the class appearing in the R-MIM diagram contains a list of the RIM attributes that are permitted to appear inside that class. Each attribute has a name. It may be required to appear, in which case an * follows the name. In a few cases, it must not use a null flavor, in which case, it will appear in bold.

Following all of this text will be a colon and then the name of the HL7 data type which is used to represent it. If the data type is any of the specializations of CD or CD itself, it will be followed by the string CWE or CNE. These two values indicate whether the value set specified is suggested (coded with extensions or CWE), or required (coded no extensions or CNE). The cardinality will appear in square brackets, indicting a lower and upper bounds. Again, if the data type is some sort of code, the concept domain, value set, or specific code used for the code is given. In CDA, this always appears following <=, but in later HL7 Version 3 messages, the = or <= symbols are used. The = symbol means that only the specified code can be used. The <= symbol means that code or any of its subtypes (or value set members) can be used.

The CDA Hierarchical Description

Of course, all of the information that appears in an HL7 Version 3 Model can also be stored and represented in tables. HL7 Version 3 specifications include what is called the Hierarchical Message Description or HMD in the standard. In CDA this is called the Hierarchical Description because CDA describes a document, not a message.

The first part of the CDA Hierarchical Description is shown in Fig. 12.6 on the next page.

Table 12.5 Columns in the CDA HD

Column	Description
Element name	The XML element name.
Card	The lower and upper bounds (* = ∞)
Mand	This column contains an M when the item is mandatory.
Conf	This column contains an R when the item is required.
Rim source	The name of the class from which the item is derived.
of Message Element Type	The data type or class name used to send the element.
Src	Indicates how this item is being defined. N – New item being defined. D – Uses an HL7 Version 3 Datatype U – Reuse of a predefined item R – Reuse of a item being defined (recursively).
Domain	Indicates the concept domain, value set, or code that is assigned to items using a coded data type.
CS	CNE (Coded No Extensions) if the domain is required or CWE (Coded With Extensions) if it is recommended.
Abst	This column contains a Y when to identify the beginning of a set of choices.
Nt	The default values for the data element.

No	Element Name	Max	Co	Rim Source	of Message Element Type	S	Domain	CS	Abst	Nt
	CDA (POCD_HD000040) Hierarchical Description									
	ClinicalDocument			Document	ClinicalDocument					
				InfrastructureRoot						
1	typeId	M	R	Act	II	N				Default: @root="2.16.840.1.113883.1.3"; @extension="POCD_H...
2	classCode	M	R	Act	CS	D	DOCCLIN	CNE		Default: DOCCLIN
3	moodCode	M	R	Act	CS	D	EVN	CNE		Default: EVN
4	id		R	Act	II	N				
5	code		R	Act	CE	D	DocumentType	CWE		
6	title			Act	ST	D				
7	effectiveTime		R	Act	TS	D				
8	confidentialityCode		R	Act	CE	D	x_BasicConfidentialityKind	CWE		
9	languageCode			Act	CS	D	HumanLanguage	CNE		Default: @codeSystem="2.16.840.1.113883.6.121"
10	setId			ContextStructure	II	D				
11	versionNumber			ContextStructure	INT	D				
12	copyTime			Document	TS	O				DesignNote: Deprecated
13	**recordTarget**			Act	SET<RecordTarget>	N				
14	typeCode	M	R	Participation	CS	D	RCT	CNE		Default: RCT
15	contextControlCode	M		Participation	CS	D	OP	CNE		Default: OP
16	**patientRole**			Participation	PatientRole	N				
17	classCode	M	R	Role	CS	D	PAT	CNE		Default: PAT
18	id			Role	SET<II>	D				
19	addr			Role	SET<AD>	D				
20	telecom			Role	SET<TEL>	D				
21	**patient**			Role	Patient	N				
22	classCode	M	R	Entity	CS	D	PSN	CNE		Default: PSN
23	determinerCode	M	R	Entity	CS	D	INSTANCE	CNE		Default: INSTANCE
24	id			Entity	II	D				DesignNote: Deprecated
25	name			Entity	SET<PN>	D				
26	administrativeGenderCode			LivingSubject	CE	D	AdministrativeGender	CWE		
27	birthTime			LivingSubject	TS	D				
28	maritalStatusCode			Person	CE	D	MaritalStatus	CWE		
29	religiousAffiliationCode			Person	CE	D	ReligiousAffiliation	CWE		
30	raceCode			Person	CE	D	Race	CWE		
31	ethnicGroupCode			Person	CE	D	Ethnicity	CWE		
32	**guardian**			Entity	SET<Guardian>	N				
33	classCode	M	R	Role	CS	D	GUARD	CNE		Default: GUARD
34	id			Role	SET<II>	D				
35	code			Role	CE	D	RoleCode	CWE		
36	addr			Role	SET<AD>	D				
37	telecom			Role	SET<TEL>	D				
38	**guardianChoice**				Person | Organization	N			Y	
39	**guardianPerson**			LivingSubject	Person	N				
40	classCode	M	R	Entity	CS	D	PSN	CNE		Default: PSN
41	determinerCode	M	R	Entity	CS	D	INSTANCE	CNE		Default: INSTANCE
42	name			Entity	SET<PN>	D				
43	*guardianOrganization*			Entity	Organization	U				
44	birthplace			Entity	Birthplace	N				

Fig. 12.6 The CDA hierarchal description

Summary

- The six backbone base classes of the RIM are Act, Participation, Role, Entity, ActRelationship, and RoleLink.
- Participation, ActRelationship and Role link are UML association classes.
- Role sometimes acts like a UML association class.
- Hungarian notation helps identify data types associated with RIM class attributes.
- Inert properties of an act cannot be negated.
- Class attributes can be mandatory, required or optional.
- Context propagation is a simplifying feature that reduces message size when information is serialized.
- The CDA Hierarchical description is a table oriented view of the CDA Information Model diagram.

Questions

1. What are the six RIM backbone classes?
2. Which backbone class is NOT used in CDA Release 2?
3. How would you identify the data type of a RIM class attribute in XML?
4. How do structural attributes differ from other class attributes in an HL7 Model?
5. Is `statusCode` a descriptive or inert property?
6. What is the different between descriptive and inert properties?
7. Assuming normal context conduction rules, if a clinical document has author A, and a section 1 of that document has author B, who is the author of a clinical statement in section 1?
8. In other sections that do not list an author?
9. In what ways could this interpretation be altered by changing other attributes in the CDA document?
10. What is the difference between *mandatory* and *required*?

Research Questions

1. How did HL7 solve the ambiguity regarding negation for the Observation class?
2. What is an example case where an Entity would use a `determinerCode` of KIND? INSTANCE?
3. What RIM class attributes have changed since CDA Release 2?

Reference

1. Charles Simonyi, <u>Hungarian Notation</u>, November 1999, Microsoft Corporation. Available on the web at http://msdn2.microsoft.com/en-us/library/aa260976(VS.60).aspx

Clinical Document Infrastructure

13

The CDA™ standard describes the structure of a clinical document using an HL7 modeling drawing that is based on UML as explained above. A miniature of that diagram appears below. This diagram is called the CDA R-MIM. In HL7 Version 3, the term R-MIM stands for restricted message information model. Of course CDA describes a document, not a message, so you will sometimes hear this described as a Restricted Meta-Information model.

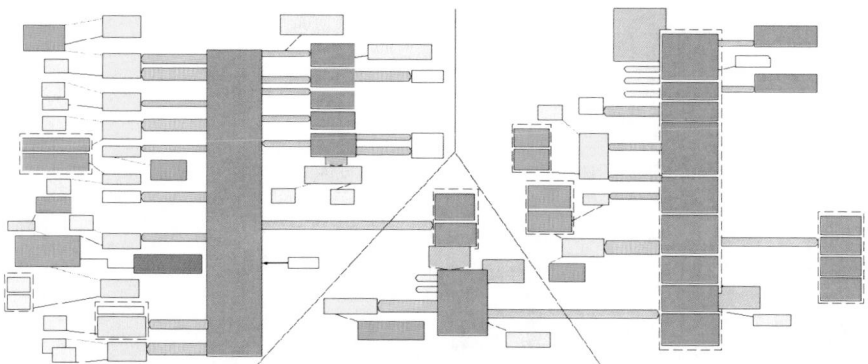

Fig. 13.1 The CDA R-MIM (This diagram and the various fragments of it that follow in Chaps. 13 through 16 appear in the HL7 Clinical Document Architecture Release 2.0 standard and are used with permission)

The CDA R-MIM diagram has three major parts, corresponding to the parts of the model related to the three different levels of the CDA specification. The CDA Header on the left hand side is described in Chap. 14 and models the CDA Level 1 content. The human readable narrative appears in the center bottom triangle in the diagram and models the CDA Level 2 content. Finally, the clinical statements on the right make up the machine readable content for CDA Level 3.

K.W. Boone, *The CDA™ Book*,
DOI: 10.1007/978-0-85729-336-7_13, © Springer-Verlag London Limited 2011

13.1
<ClinicalDocument>

The <ClinicalDocument> element is the root XML element in all CDA documents. This element typically contains all of the namespace declarations necessary for the clinical document; may declare the realm for which the document was written; always indicates the version of CDA in use; and may declare the business rules that this document asserts conformance to. An example <ClinicalDocument> element implementing all of these features is shown in the figure below.

```
<ClinicalDocument xmlns='urn:hl7-org:v3'
   xmlns:xsi='http://www.w3.org/2001/XMLSchema-instance'
   classCode='DOCCLIN' moodCode='EVN'
>
   <realmCode code='…'/>
   <typeId root='2.16.840.1.113883.1.3'
      extension='POCD_HD000040'/>
   <templateId root='2.16.840.1.113883.10.20.1'/>
         :
</ClinicalDocument>
```

Fig. 13.2 ClinicalDocument example

Namespace Declarations

There are two namespace declarations commonly used in the CDA XML representation. See Sect. 4.2 for more details on how namespaces are used in XML markup.

Namespace	Prefix	Description
urn:hl7-org:v3	*Default*	This namespace declaration is needed in all HL7 Version 3 specifications, including the CDA. I recommend using it as the default namespace because it makes for easier to read CDA instances.
http://www.w3.org/2001/ XMLSchema-instance	xsi	This namespace is needed to declare the data types used by the <value> elements that appear within <observation> elements or to override the default data type used in the CDA schemas.

classCode='DOCCLIN'

In HL7 Version 3 XML representations, the classCode XML attribute indicates which RIM class is being represented in the XML. The <ClinicalDocument> element always represents an instance of the clinical document act in the RIM, so the CDA schema gives this XML attribute a fixed value of `DOCCLIN` in the schema. Some CDA documents will contain this XML attribute in the `<ClinicalDocument>` element and others will not. It can safely be ignored during processing.

moodCode='EVN'

The mood of an act in HL7 Version 3 describes both its placement in time, and the way it is used in clinical statements. This borrows from the linguistic concept of mood for inflecting a verb. The `<ClinicalDocument>` element always represents an act that has occurred, and so the `moodCode` attribute is set by the CDA schema to the fixed value `EVN`. Some CDA documents will contain this XML attribute in the `<ClinicalDocument>` and others will not. It can safely be ignored during processing.

13.2
Infrastructure Elements

Infrastructure elements are so named because they are part of the XML infrastructure used with CDA. They appear because of requirements in the XML Implementation Technology Specification that are common to all XML representations in HL7 Version 3, not just those using CDA. These XML elements can appear on any RIM class appearing in a CDA document, not just the `<ClinicalDocument>` element. They always appear first in these XML elements, and in the order given below.

<realmCode>

The `<realmCode>` element is optional. When it appears, it declares the realm (or realms, as it can repeat) for which the content is written. The realm code is often used to indicate which regional policies are applicable to the content. Many HL7 implementation guides are written for the "Universal Realm"; whose `code` is `UV`. Others, such as the Continuity of Care Document Implementation Guide, are specified for a country specific realm (i.e., for CCD, the US realm).

Inside a CDA document, the realm code acts as a declaration of the target audience for the content and indicates the regional policies which have been applied. The bodies governing the realms are the HL7 Affiliates in each country. For example, HL7 Canada is the authority on the CA realm. At the time of publication, HL7 still did not have a US Affiliate, and so the US realm is governed by HL7 International.

<typeId>

The `<typeId>` element identifies the version of the HL7 standard model being represented in the XML. Since there is only one model that is being represented, there can be only one `<typeId>` element. While many XML based standards represent the model and version information in the namespace for the XML, HL7 Version 3 is a bit different. HL7 Version 3 components can be defined in different standards and mixed and matched. This requires versioning to be done differently. The `<typeId>` element serves this purpose.

The `<ClinicalDocument>` element of the CDA requires a `<typeId>` element. This `<typeId>` element uses fixed values for the `root` and `extension` XML attributes. These values are shown in the example above.

The `<typeId>` element may appear on other XML elements representing a RIM class in the CDA, but is not required. This could be done to indicate that the XML element also conforms to an HL7 standard model identified in some other specification. This is allowed but entirely uncommon in CDA Release 2.0 implementations. In CDA Release 3 this XML element should be more common.

\<templateId\>

The `<templateId>` element identifies a template which has been applied to the XML element in which it appears. Essentially a template is an identified set of business rules. The ability to associate business rules with the XML in CDA has proven to be extremely powerful, and so has become one of the most important infrastructure elements in the CDA standard.

Chapter 19 on Templates describes how CDA uses templates in more detail. More than one `<templateId>` element can appear on the XML representation of one of the RIM classes. The existence of a `<templateId>` element is an assertion of conformance to the business rules which are specified in the template it identifies. This element may and often does repeat because multiple sets of business rules can be applied to a single RIM class.

Summary

- The CDA R-MIM diagram describes the structure of the content in the CDA standard.
- The 3 CDA Levels correspond to the CDA Header, coded sections in the CDA body, and clinical statements.
- The `<realmCode>`, `<typeId>` and `<templateId>` elements can appear in any RIM class in the XML of a CDA document.
- The `<templateId>` element is one of the most important infrastructure elements in CDA implementations.

Questions

1. Why can the `classCode` and `moodCode` XML attributes of the `<ClinicalDocument>` element be safely ignored?
2. Where can infrastructure elements appear in a CDA document?

3. Which infrastructure element must be used in a CDA document and where must it appear?
4. Which infrastructure attribute cannot repeat?

_____

Research Questions

1. Select a CDA implementation guide suitable for your realm. What `<realmCode>` and `<templateId>` elements does it require for the document?
2. What was the first CDA implementation guide to use `<templateId>`?

The CDA™ Header

14

The CDA header is the first part of the CDA Document. It includes all content up to the `<component>` element that contains the body of the document. The CDA header sets the context (see page 13) for the content of the clinical document.

```
<ClinicalDocument xmlns='urn:hl7-org:v3'
    xmlns:xsi='http://www.w3.org/2001/XMLSchema-instance'
    classCode='DOCCLIN' moodCode='EVN'
>
    <realmCode code='...'/>
    <typeId root='2.16.840.1.113883.1.3'
        extension='POCD_HD000040'/>
    <templateId root=' 2.16.840.1.113883.10.20.1'/>
    <id root='...' extension='...'/>
    <code code='...' displayName='...'
        codeSystem='...' codeSystemName='...'/>
    <title>...</title>
    <effectiveTime value='...'/>
    <confidentialityCode code='...' displayName='...'
        codeSystem='...' codeSystemName='...'/>
    <languageCode code='...'/>
    <setId root='...' extension='...'/>
    <versionNumber value='...'/>
    <copyTime value='...'/>
        :
</ClinicalDocument>
```

Fig. 14.1 CDA header example

The CDA header is made up of three different kinds of elements, in the following order.

1. RIM Attributes of the `ClinicalDocument` class
2. Participants attached to the `ClinicalDocument` class
3. Related acts connected to the `ClinicalDocument` class.

The RIM attributes appear in the order in which they appear on the CDA R-MIM. The participants and related acts appear in an order predefined by the XML ITS and the HL7 tools which were used to develop the CDA standard.

K.W. Boone, *The CDA™ Book*,
DOI: 10.1007/978-0-85729-336-7_14, © Springer-Verlag London Limited 2011

14.1
Clinical Document RIM Attributes

The RIM attributes of the ClinicalDocument class are shown in the figure below, which comes from the CDA R-MIM.

Fig. 14.2 The
ClinicalDocument class

clinicalDocument

classCode* : <= DOCCLIN
moodCode* : <= EVN
id*: II [1..1]
code*: CE CWE [1..1] <= DocumentType
title: ST [0..1]
effectiveTime*: TS [1..1]
confidentialityCode*: CE CWE [1..1]
 <= x_BasicConfidentialityKind
languageCode: CS CNE [0..1] <= HumanLanguage
setId: II [0..1]
versionNumber: INT [0..1]
copyTime: TS [0..1] (Deprecated)

The class attributes associated with the ClinicalDocument class identify the document, describe what is inside it, indicate relevant dates and times, and help decide which policies should be applied to it with respect to patient privacy.

Document Identity

The id, setId and versionNumber class attributes are used to identify the clinical document. The id class attribute provides a single unique identity for the clinical document. Two documents with the same id recorded inside must in fact be identical with respect to content. The bytes used to represent the XML could be different (e.g., one stored in EBCDIC and the other in UCS-16), but the content must be the same.

Each clinical document describes a set of care events occurring during an episode of care. It usually requires only one edition describe these events in a clinical document. There are cases, however, where a document needs to be revised.

Describing the Document

The code and title class attributes serve the same purpose for different audiences. The code class attribute describes the type of the clinical document using a coded value suitable for machine interpretation. The title class attribute provides a string suitable for human interpretation. The intent of title is to be a human readable common name for the document, e.g., History and Physical Note, or Discharge Summary, describing the type of service described in the document. *That means that title, if present, must be included in the human readable rendering of the CDA content.*

You will note that the `title` class attribute is optional. I strongly recommend its use in all clinical documents. That is because the title is what will most often be displayed in user interfaces showing collections of clinical documents.

The use of both a `title` and `code` attribute is a pattern you will also see again in sections. There is a great deal of benefit to separating the machine readable codes from the human readable titles. One of these is that it allows legacy document titles to remain unaltered when new systems are put into place. This benefits the users of those new systems who may be reassured that the content they expected is still present. It also allows automated systems to process that content by allowing for a coded value. The two separate components allow the best of both worlds without making the human users conform to the needs of the automated system.

The `title` is an optional component of the clinical document but the `code` is not. When generating clinical documents, there is no real reason to omit the title because a human readable title can at the very least be determined from the human readable display name associated with the document code. Therefore, I strongly recommend that every clinical document contain a title.

Coding a CDA Document

While a CDA document can be described using any code system, the preferred set of codes comes from the LOINC® vocabulary. LOINC® stands for Logical Observation Identifiers and Codes and is produced by the Regeinstrief Institute. The full set of LOINC® codes can be freely obtained from http://www.loinc.org, along with a program called RELMA which can be used to search for LOINC® codes. LOINC® can also be searched for online.

Originally started as a vocabulary to identify laboratory test codes, LOINC® has long since expanded into other clinical areas. One of these has been the development of a methodology for creating codes for documents and the establishment of numerous document codes.

LOINC® classifies documents on four main axes: Type of document, type of service described, kind of author and location of service provided. Types of documents used in healthcare include those that are specific to a patient and those with other subjects of interest. Among the patient specific documents for which CDA is well suited, are those that provide documentation of care (a history and physical note), administrative documents (e.g., an explanation of benefits form), case reports (e.g., an adverse event report) and legal documents (e.g., consent for a procedure or to release information). Other kinds of documents which LOINC® can provide codes for include order sets, clinical guidelines and drug package inserts. There are some CDA-like document standards in HL7 that can support a few of these document types. Most document type codes found in LOINC are those describing documentation of care.

LOINC® includes codes for documentation of the most common services provided by healthcare providers. These include History and Physicals, Consultations, Operations and Procedures, Discharge and Transfer, Progress notes, laboratory reports and imaging studies.

LOINC® often provides very detailed codes which pre-coordinate the type of document and service with the professional level of the provider (e.g., Physician, Resident or Nurse), and the location of service (e.g., Hospital, Home Care, Long Term Care, Emergency Department or Ambulatory Care). The CDA standard provides other locations for documenting this level of detail. The professional level of the provider of the service can be stored in the code of the performer or author role. The setting where care was provided can be coded in the location participation class of the encompassingEncounter act.

This means that there are often two or more different ways to code the same document. Take for example the code 34106-5 which is a Physician Hospital Discharge Summary, and the code 28574-2 which is a Discharge Summary where the provider level and location are unspecified. Either of these codes could be used for a Discharge Summary that was produced by an attending physician at a hospital.

Which is the best code to use? The HL7 Structured Documents workgroup shows a distinct preference for the least restrictive code (28574-2) for a number of reasons. First of all, it makes it easier to find documents by the type of service performed if only one code is used for the same service, independent of location or professional level of the performer or author. Imagine trying to discover all notes for a given service only to discover that you missed one because you were not aware of all the possible codes that could be used for that service (there are 11 for Discharge Summary). That would be frustrating at the very least, and could be catastrophic at the very worst.

Other Document Descriptors

The languageCode class attribute describes the primary language of the clinical document. This may be reported in a single languageCode element using the CE data type. The set of codes used for languages in HL7 is the same set of codes that are used to report language on the web. These are described in detail in RFC-3066 [1] and use the ISO-639 [2] language codes and ISO-3166 [3] country codes.

Note that ISO-3166 has three parts. Part 1 includes country codes and part 3 includes codes that were formerly used for countries. The language tags used in HL7 Version 3 should accept languages made up of content from both part 1 and part 3. Part 2 includes country subdivisions (e.g., States, Provinces and Territories) and is not typically used in language codes.

Date and Time

The effectiveTime class attribute indicates the creation time of the clinical document. More accurately, CDA Release 2 defines the effective time of a clinical document to be the time when it was created, which is not entirely correct. The effective time of a clinical document is the time between its release for care, and the time when it is withdrawn from use or no longer valid for care. In almost all cases, this latter value is never known in advance, and certainly never known with 100% certainty because a document can be revised and rereleased (with a new identifier) replacing a prior version at any time. The creation time of a clinical document should match the earliest participation time of all of the authors of the clinical document.

The copyTime class attribute is a holdover from CDA Release 1.0 and should not be used; it was deprecated in CDA Release 2.0. In CDA Release 1.0 this was intended to capture the first time the CDA document was copied, printed or otherwise released for care. This is really document management metadata, and not something that the application creating a CDA document could be expected to know.

Confidentiality

A great deal of attention is paid to confidentiality of information in clinical care. However, rules about how documents are to be treated with regard to confidentiality are subject to change according to patient consent, local policies, and regulation and law.

CDA Release 2.0 supports the capture of one and only one code to describe the sensitivity of the document content. It is unfortunately captured in a class attribute called the confidentialityCode. The implication is that this class attribute describes the confidentiality policy requirements. The reality is that the value set recommended for CDA simply describes the sensitivity of the information.

It anticipates that confidentiality is described in levels, from least to most restricted, much like document classification levels of secret, top secret, and eyes only in spy movies. The recommended value set for CDA has three values, Normal, Restricted, and Very Restricted. My recommendation is to stick with this set, or use a similar set.

Since the release of CDA Release 2.0, additional values have been added to the HL7 Vocabulary for confidentiality to address multiple axes around which policy around confidentiality can be created (e.g., sexual activity, disease carrier status, alcohol and substance abuse). This is not a good idea because it exposes the reason why a document was made restricted access. Codes like these that are too specific to policy also expose the policies that make a document sensitive, and therefore the kind of information present in them.

You should also understand that this was the level of sensitivity at the time the document was published. Policy can change unpredictably, but a CDA document once written is immutable. Therefore it can only report what is known about policy at the time it is created. You must provide metadata outside of the document to support management of access controls based on these kinds of policies.

If you are generating a CDA Release 2.0 document and do not know what to put in this required field, the best choice is to use the HL7 suggested vocabulary, and the code "N" to indicate Normal confidentiality, as shown in the figure below.

```
<confidentialityCode code='N' displayName='Normal'
    codeSystem='2.16.840.1.113883.5.25'
    codeSystemName='Confidentiality'
/>
```

Fig. 14.3 Reporting confidentialityCode

Note that documents are at least as sensitive as the most sensitive data element that is contained within them, but could be more so depending upon what facts are revealed by the combination of data contained within the document. To use a common example, knowing just date of birth, or zip or postal code, or gender is usually not enough to identity an individual (But not always: There are a few residential zip codes (e.g., 20500) that readily identify very small groups of individuals.). However, the three components together can be enough to identify a single person [4].

14.2
Acts

There are several acts related to the CDA document that can also be tracked in the CDA Header, and further contribute to the document's context. These include information about prior (related) documents, the specific services performed, the encounter in which they took place, the orders related to the document and the consents provided by the patient associated with these services.

Related Documents

Documents can be replaced (RPLC), added to (APND) or created by transforming (XFRM) other documents. Transformations can be automated (e.g., from the CDA XML to Portable Document Format), or manual (e.g., abstracting). The CDA standard allows these relationships to be recorded using the relatedDocument *clone* of the act relationship, and the details of the related document to be recorded in the parentDocument class.

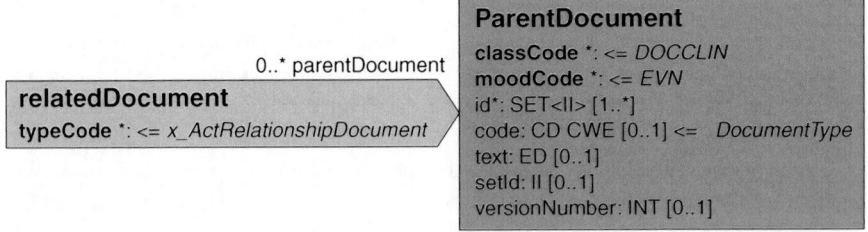

Fig. 14.4 The relatedDocument association and ParentDocument class

The type of relationship appears in the typeCode class attribute of the relatedDocument class. There are limits on the number and types of relationships that can appear. A CDA document can report only one predecessor document of which it is a transform, addition, or replacement. Thus, a single document cannot replace, be an addenda to, or transformation of two or more other documents. It also cannot be simultaneously a replacement for one document and addenda to another. It could be a transformation of one document that is an addenda or replacement for another, but that is as complex as the CDA standard allows.

The examples below show the XML used in replacement, addenda and transformation use cases.

```
<relatedDocument typeCode='REPL'>
    <parentDocument>
        <id root='...' extension='...'/>
    </parentDocument>
</relatedDocument>
```

Fig. 14.5 Use of relatedDocument to indicate replacement

```
<relatedDocument typeCode='APND'>
    <parentDocument>
        <id root='...' extension='...'/>
    </parentDocument>
</relatedDocument>
```

Fig. 14.6 Use of relatedDocument to indicate addenda

```
<relatedDocument typeCode='XFRM'>
    <parentDocument>
        <id root='...' extension='...'/>
    </parentDocument>
</relatedDocument>
```

Fig. 14.7 Use of relatedDocument to indicate transformation

One could imagine producing a summary document by transformation of all documents related to a particular episode. The CDA standard does not prevent this from being done, but it does prevent all the source documents from being recorded in the parentDocument class. Fortunately, in this case, you can record the documents that are the sources of information in references described in the chapters that follow.

The Parent Document

The parent document is a prior documentation event, so the classCode and moodCode are fixed by the CDA standard to DOCCLIN and EVN respectively. The identity of the document is the very least that must be transmitted in the id class attribute (and possibly the setId and versionNumber attributes).

A reference to the parent document can be transmitted in the text attribute. While this attribute is of the ED data type (see page 9), it is restricted by the CDA standard to allow only links to the content to be provided in a `<reference>` element. This is one of those constraints on CDA that are not addressed in the CDA Schema.

Services

Each CDA documents a variety of different services performed for the patient. These services can be described at a very high level (e.g., History and Physical or Consultation), or at greater levels of granularity (history taking, detailed physical examination, immunizations given, etc.).

Fig. 14.8 The documentationOf association and ServiceEvent class

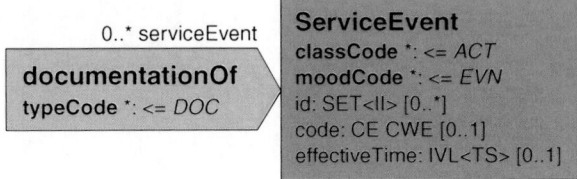

The `documentationOf` relationship is fully specified by the CDA standard. The details will appear in the `serviceEvent` class or the `performer` association attached to it.

The `classCode` class attribute in the `serviceEvent` class can be any kind of act that can be represented in the HL7 Act class hierarchy, an encounter, a procedure, an observation (e.g., a diagnostic study), etc. This is the service event that the CDA document is describing.

Some document types restrict the service event to just one event, that being the most important event being addressed in the document. The HL7 Continuity of Care Document Implementation Guide (CCD) describes one such document. A CCD is intended to describe care provided over a period of time, and so restricts the cardinality and content of the `serviceEvent`.

The HL7 Continuity of Care Document Implementation Guide (CCD) requires that `classCode` be set to PCPR, which is provision of care. That is because CCD is essentially a snapshot of the patient summary data created as a result of any sort of care provided over a period of time.

```
<documentationOf>
   <serviceEvent classCode='PCPR'>
      <effectiveTime>
         <low value='…'/>
         <high value='…'/>
      </effectiveTime>
   </serviceEvent>
</documentationOf>
```

Fig. 14.9 ServiceEvent example

The `code` class attribute of the service event provides more detail. It is commonly completed using some sort of procedure code (e.g. CPT, ICD-9-CM Procedures, or descending from the SNOMED CT Procedure hierarchy) to describe the event being documented. However, it could also be an order code for a laboratory test when the CDA document is used to deliver lab results.

The `effectiveTime` class attribute represents the clinically effective time of the service event. It does not necessarily include all the time that is involved in the preparation, etc. (that be captured in the RIM `activityTime` class attribute if it were permitted). Again, using CCD as an example, the `effectiveTime` class attribute captures the time span over which the care that is documented in the CCD was provided. In a discharge summary, this same class attribute would normally record the entire length of stay as the `effectiveTime`, since a discharge summary provides an overview of what happened over the course of an inpatient stay.

A CDA document can provide documentation of any number of service events (if the business rules for the document allow it). In most cases, every Act provided in the CDA document is some sort of service event. Some would wonder why `serviceEvent` even exists then, since this appears to be an alternate way of stating the same information in the standard.

Healthcare applications that use unstructured narrative will often have the service codes associated with that narrative. Putting `serviceEvent` in the CDA header allows these applications to describe the services performed without requiring them to use the CDA narrative XML format.

The `serviceEvent` classes that are found in the CDA Header are also expected to be significant (in the eye of the beholder) events relevant to application workflows. These may be events that need to be billed for, or to supply a record of certain clinical activities, such as medication reconciliation. Putting this information in the header makes it quickly accessible for application processing. Note though, that these uses are often based on local business rules for the system generating the CDA documents. There is relatively little established best-practice on use of `serviceEvent`, and the level of detail to which it should be completed.

Performers

Each service event is performed by one or more persons acting in some sort of role assigned by the healthcare provider organization. This is demonstrated in the figure below.

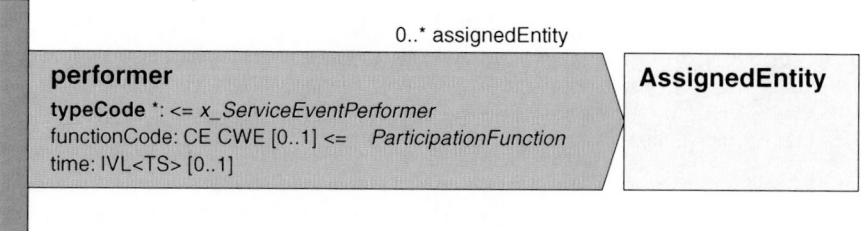

Fig. 14.10 Service Event performers

CDA permits the identification of the performer (PRF), and you can also distinguish further between primary performer (PPRF) and secondary performers (SPRF) in the typeCode class attribute. The function being performed by the performer is described in the functionCode class attribute, and the time over which they performed that function may appear in the time class attribute. The functionCode class attribute describes the functional role of the performer. See page 113 for a more detailed description of functional and structural roles.

The example below shows the XML used to represent the performer in a service event in a CDA document.

```
<performer typeCode='PRF'>
   <functionCode code='…' codeSystem='…'
         codeSystemName='…' displayName='…'/>
   <time>
       <low value='…'/>
       <high value='…'/>
   </time>
   <assignedEntity>
       <id extension='…' root='…'/>
       <code code='…' codeSystem='…'
         codeSystemName='…' displayName='…'/>
   </assignedEntity>
</performer>
```

Fig. 14.11 Performer participation example

Orders

A CDA document can be produced as the result of a service that was ordered. For example, when an imaging study, lab test or referral are requested, the results can be returned using the CDA standard. Healthcare workflows want to be able to link results back to the order that requested them, so the CDA model allows these to be recorded.

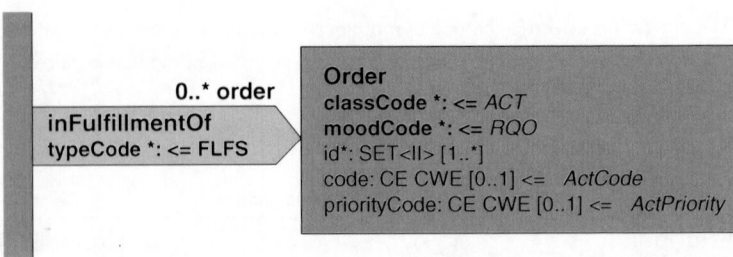

Fig. 14.12 The inFulfillmentOf association and order class

The inFulfillmentOf association links the document to the order that eventually resulted in the creation of the document. That association is fully specified by the CDA standard. The details of the order appear in the `order` class. The order requires at least one order identifier. This identifier can be the order identifier produced by the placer of the order, or the filler of the order, or both can be provided. Best practice is to include both if you have them.

The `code` class attribute of the `order` class will indicate what service was requested, e.g., the lab test, imaging procedure, or type of encounter. This class attribute also should be provided when known.

Finally, the `priorityCode` class attribute indicates the priority of the order (e.g., STAT, as soon as possible, routine). This code can be used by receivers to determine how to alert providers that the document has been received.

The example below shows the `infulfillmentOf` association being used to identify the order number and type of order that was placed. This order is being fulfilled by the CDA document in which it appears.

```
<infulfillmentOf>
    <order>
        <id root='…' extension='…'/>
        <code code='…' codeSystem='…'
            codeSystemName='…' displayName='…'/>
    </order>
</infulfillmentOf>
```

Fig. 14.13 infulfillmentOf example

Consents

A CDA documents a particular service being performed. In many cases, providers of these services are required to obtain informed consent of the patient before performing those services.

Fig. 14.14 authorization association and consent class

The authorization association class is fully defined by CDA and links the document to the consents given. The `consent` class allows providers to document that an informed consent was obtained, and to indicate what type of consent was provided.

At the very minimum, the `consent` class simply indicates that consent was obtained, and provides no further details. The `id` class attribute can be populated to indicate any identifier associated with the consent (e.g., the identifier of the signed consent form). The `code` class attribute allows the type of consent obtained to be documented.

```
<authorization>
    <consent>
        <id root='…' extension='…'/>
        <code code='…' codeSystem='…'
            codeSystemName='…' displayName='…'/>
        <statusCode code='completed'/>
    </consent>
</authorization>
```

Fig. 14.15 Authorization example

Encounter

The service events documented in a CDA instance are usually provided as part of a clinical encounter. The model for the encounter is shown in the figure below.

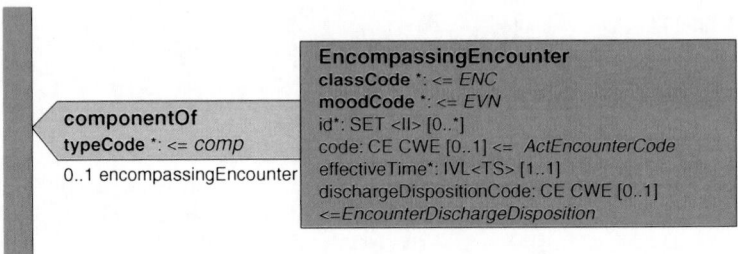

Fig. 14.16 componentOf association and encompassingEncounter class

The `componentOf` association links the document to the encounter it documents and is fully specified by the CDA standard. The `encompassingEncounter` class describes the encounter event.

The `effectiveTime` class attribute is required and describes the time of the encounter. This uses the IVL_TS data type so that the duration of the encounter can be captured.

The identifier and type of encounter are captured in the `id` and `code` class attributes respectively. The encounter identifier is variously known as the visit id, encounter id, appointment id, or sometimes even the account number[1] in different healthcare settings.

---

[1] The patient account number is usually a billing related identifier associated with a specific patient stay, but identifies the patient account rather than the visit itself. However, not everyone assigns a visit identifier in their workflows.

The code class attribute typically identifies the type of encounter. In the US these would typically be recorded using something like the CPT-4 Evaluation and Management codes. They can also be described using the HL7 ActEncounterCode vocabulary, which provides a very high level description of the type of encounter, or using vocabularies like SNOMED CT. The dischargeDisposition class attribute indicates what happened to the patient after the encounter was completed. This often indicates whether the patient was discharged to home, transferred to another facility, or admitted.

The figure below shows the XML used to represent the componentOf association.

```
<componentOf>
    <encompassingEncounter>
        <id root='…' extension='…'/>
        <code code='…' codeSystem='…'
            codeSystemName='…' displayName='…'/>
        <statusCode code='completed'/>
        <effectiveTime>
            <low value='…'/>
            <high value='…'/>
        </effectiveTime>
        <dischargeDispositionCode code='…' codeSystem='…'
            codeSystemName='…' displayName='…'/>
    </encompassingEncounter>
</componentOf>
```

Fig. 14.17 encompassingEncounter example

Also associated with the encounter are the encounter location, and the various parties involved in the encounter.

Encounter Location

The model for encounter location is depicted below.

The location association is fully specified by the CDA standard. The healthcareFacility class uses the id and code class attributes to indicate an

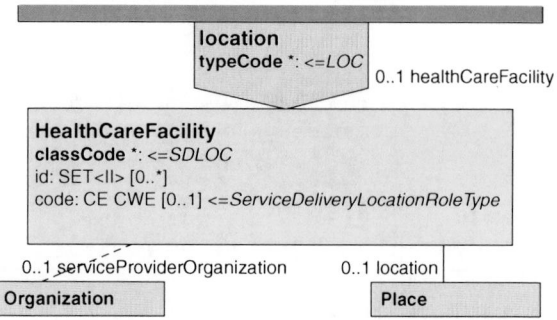

Fig. 14.18 location association and healthCareFacility class

identifier associated with the facility, and to describe the type of facility. The place class gives the address of the location and is the *player* of the location role. The organization class is the *scoper* of the location role. In an organization with multiple facilities, a specific facility could be the location, while the organization would scope that location. When there is only one facility associated with an organization the address of the organization and the address of the location are identical. Since neither of these classes is required, implementations can choose to use one or the other to record location details.

The choice of where to put this should depend upon how the implementation expects the receiver to make use of this data. A common use case for facility location data is to be able to contact individuals at that specific location. In that use case, the organization class can supply both the address and contact information like phone numbers. The example below shows the XML used to represent a location containing both an organization and a place.

Note that in the following, the id and code class attributes of the healthcareFacility class will often be different from the id and standardIndustryClassCode class attributes appearing in the serviceProviderOrganization class. The service provider organization may simply be classified as a "healthcare provider organization", whereas the specific facility where care is provided could be classified as an urgent care center, a hospital, or an outpatient clinic. Similarly, their identifiers would be related to the role (of the healthcareFacility) and the identity of the service provider organization. The former might be a mandated identifier used to track healthcare provider organizations (e.g., the National Provider ID as used in the US), while the latter could be an identifier of the organization, such as a tax ID number.

```xml
<location>
    <healthcareFacility>
        <id root='…' extension='…'/>
        <code code='…' codeSystem='…'
            codeSystemName='…' displayName='…'/>
        <location>
            <name>…</name>
            <addr>…</addr>
        </location>
        <serviceProviderOrganization>
            <id root='…' extension='…'/>
            <name>…</name>
            <telecom value='…'/>
            <addr>…</addr>
            <standardIndustryClassCode code='…'
                codeSystem='…' codeSystemName='…'
                displayName='…'/>
        </serviceProviderOrganization>
    </healthcareFacility>
</location>
```

Fig. 14.19 Location example

Encounter Participants

Participants in the encounter include the responsible party and others that may have participated in the encounter. The HL7 value set allowed for the other participants is shown in the table below.

Table 14.1 Encounter participants

Code	Print name	Description
ADM	Admitter	The healthcare provider responsible for admitting the patient.
ATND	Attender	The healthcare provider responsible for the patient's care during the admission.
CON	Consultant	A healthcare provider that advises on particular aspects of care.
DIS	Discharger	The healthcare provider responsible for discharging the patient.
REF	Referring	The person (usually but not always a healthcare provider) who referred the patient for care.

Contents of this table are drawn from the HL7 Vocabulary Standard with permission. Columns 1 and 2 come directly from the standard. Column 3 is the authors interpretation

Fig. 14.20 Encounter participations

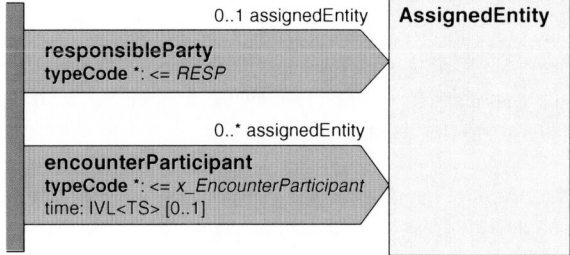

The responsible party is described in the HL7 ParticipationType vocabulary as being the person or organization with the primary responsibility for the act, in this case the encounter. Determining who the responsible party is for an encounter is determined greatly by policy. Since this responsibility is for the encounter, time of participation is not included in the participation association as it is for other encounter participants. That is because responsibility is assumed to be for the entire encounter. Thus, the participation time of the responsible party is the same as the effective time interval for the encounter.

For a typical outpatient encounter, the responsible party be the healthcare provider that the patient saw, but it could also be a provider responsible for their actions. My children most often see a nurse practitioner, but she is supervised by a pediatrician, and so he might be considered the responsible party. In an inpatient stay, this would most commonly be the patient's attending physician. In other types of clinical documents, the person responsible for the encounter might vary. For a laboratory report, this might be the director of the lab where the report was generated, but another in other diagnostic tests, it might be the healthcare provider who interprets the results, or the person responsible for supervising their work. Again, policy determines who has the final responsibility.

The example below shows the XML for the responsible party and the encounterParticipant. See Fig. 14.28 below for the XML for the assignedEntity. Note that the `typeCode` XML attribute must be specified on the `<encounterParticipant>` element.

```
<responsibleParty>
   <assignedEntity>…</assignedEntity>
</responsibleParty>
<encounterParticipant typeCode='ATND'>
   <time><low value='…'/><high value='…'/></time>
   <assignedEntity>…</assignedEntity>
</encounterParticipant>
```

Fig. 14.21 responsibleParty and encounterParticipant example

14.3
Participations and Roles in the Document Context

The context of the document includes a number of different participants in creating the document. These participations include people, organizations, and even medical devices or applications that might be responsible for creating the document. Each of these participations associates the document to a role.

The participation associations are grouped with the role classes in this section because the two parts work together. The participation association describes the *functional role*, and the role class describes the *structural role*. See the discussion of functional and structural roles found on page 113.

This section will describe these participants, including the patient, the author, data enterer, information providers, the organization maintaining a true and accurate copy of it, recipients of the document, the provider signing it, and a number of other optional participants.

Common Class Attributes for Participations

Participations in the HL7 RIM can have an associated time of participation in the `time` attribute, a signature associated with the participation, a specific function being performed as described by the `functionCode` attribute.

They can also include a code describing the awareness of the participant of their role in the act in the `awarenessCode` class attribute. Another code describes the mode of the participation (e.g., in person or remote, written communication or by telephone, etc.) using the `modeCode` class attribute.

In the CDA standard, some of these class attributes are present and in other cases they are not. In the cases where these class attributes are missing, it is because the attribute is either implied by the relationship, or is not necessary in the context of the clinical document. For example, the custodian of a clinical document is expected to be in that role for as long as it has a responsibility (determined by policy) to do so, and it would not be possible to determine what the time frame might be.

Common Class Attributes for Roles

In CDA, addresses and phone numbers are associated with people based on their roles, and appear in the `addr` and `telecom` class attributes. The reason for this distinction is because the address used by a person depends upon the role they are playing. For example, I'd give my healthcare provider my personal e-mail address before I would give them my work e-mail address, because that address is more appropriate for provider to patient communications. In just the same way, the address of my current place of residence might be used in my patient role, but my home address might be used in my role as the payer for the encounter.

Identifiers are also associated with roles, especially when the player of the role is a person (there are few people in this world who have an identifier associated with their person that is unscoped by any role relationship). Identifiers are recorded in the `id` class attribute. If you look in your wallet, you will find a number of ID cards. Each of these cards has a number on it that identifies you in the context of a specific role. If you have a drivers license, that identifies you (the player of the role) as a legal driver in a particular jurisdiction (the scoper of that role). A credit card identifies you (the player of the role) as being authorized to use the funds of a creditor (the scoper of the role) to complete a financial transaction. Similarly, the role identifiers in the CDA document uniquely identify the roles played by the various parties.

The Patient

The patient is arguably the most important person associated with the clinical document. The participation association and role classes appear in the diagram below. You should note that every CDA document requires at least one patient.

One would expect the patient to be identified in the CDA model using a participation named patient, but recall that clinical documents typically appear within a medical record.

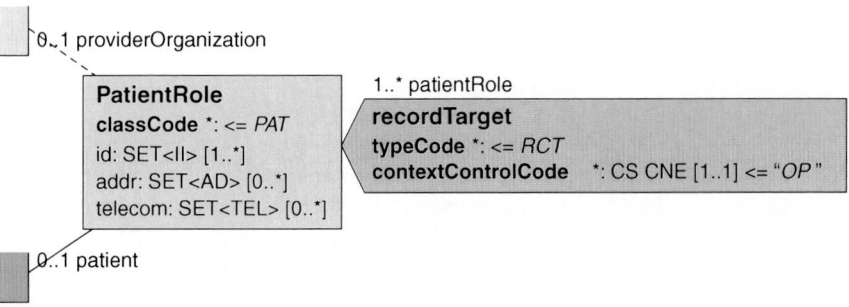

Fig. 14.22 recordTarget association and patientRole classes

The name of the participation association class is `recordTarget` because it identifies the medical record in which this document appears.

A single clinical document can appear in more than one medical record, and so more than one `recordTarget` association can be present. While uncommon, some of the use cases for this include delivery of a newborn, where the labor and delivery record would appear in both the mother and the baby's medical record, or for group therapy.

The Patient Role

The `patientRole` class in the above diagram represents the person playing the role of patient, as described in the `patient` entity class described in more detail in the next section. The patient plays this role through a provider organization, which can be described in the `providerOrganization` class. In their role as a patient, this person has at least identifier found in the id class attribute of the `patientRole` class. This is typically the medical record number of the patient, but sometimes other identifiers are included instead of or in addition to the medical record number.

The `addr` and `telecom` class attributes of the `patientRole` class represent the address and telephone numbers (or e-mail or other telecommunications addresses) used by this person in their role as patient.

The patient is assumed to be in that role at least for the duration of the encounter described by the clinical document, so the `time` attribute is omitted in this participation.

```
<recordTarget>
   <patientRole>
       <id root='…' extension='…'/>
       <addr>…</addr>
       <telecom value='…'/>
       <patient>…</patient>
       <providerOrganization>…</providerOrganization>
   </patientRole>
</recordTarget>
```

Fig. 14.23 recordTarget and patientRole XML example

The Author

The author of a clinical document can either be a person or a device.

Authors represent the first of three different kinds of information sources from the HL7 RIM that appear in the CDA, and is arguably the most important since there must be at least one author in a CDA instance. Authors create information in the clinical document based on their knowledge or application of skills. Information provided to them by other parties (see Sect. 14.3.6 below) may or may not be included in a clinical document based on the judgment of the author.

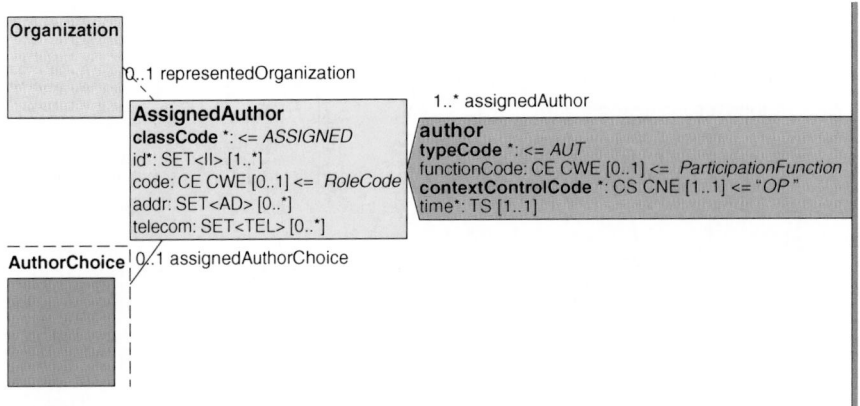

Fig. 14.24 The author participation association and assignedAuthor class

The `functionCode` attribute of the author participation class indicates the functional role of the author. The HL7 suggested vocabulary is ParticipationFunction, and appears below.

Table 14.2 Suggested functional roles for authors

Code	Description	Code	Description
ADMPHYS	Admitting physician	NASST	Nurse assistant
ANEST	Anesthetist	PCP	Primary care Physician
ANRS	Anesthesia nurse	PRISURG	Primary surgeon
ATTPHYS	Attending physician	RNDPHYS	Rounding physician
DISPHYS	Discharging physician	SASST	Second assistant Surgeon
FASST	First assistant Surgeon	SNRS	Scrub nurse
MDWF	Midwife	TASST	Third assistant

This vocabulary is recommended, but not required by the CDA standard. Other vocabularies may be used as required by local policies. A few of the possible functional roles missing from this vocabulary include consulting physician, interpreting physician (e.g., a reading radiologist) and therapist.

The `time` class attribute indicates the time at which the person or device started their participation as an author, as that may have clinical relevance.

The Assigned Author Role

The author participation associates someone or some device in the assigned role as a document author. According to the HL7 RIM, assigned roles are those where the focus is on the functional role of the player of the role rather than on their structural role.

The id class attribute identifies the author and is often connected in some way, but not the same value as the identifier used by authoring persons to access the system creating the document.

The code class attribute on the author role can be used to specify the level of education of the healthcare provider (e.g., MD, DO, PharmD, RN, or LPN) or their clinical specialty or both. CDA Release 2 recommends the use of HL7 RoleCode for vocabulary, but that can be misleading. At the time that CDA Release 2 was published, a standard could specify a concept domain, vocabulary, or value set for use with any class attribute using the Concept Descriptor data type.

The addr and telecom class attributes of the assignedAuthor class represent the address and telephone numbers (or e-mail or other telecommunications addresses) used by this person (or device) in their role as an author.

The examples below show how a person and device author might be represented in the CDA XML.

```
<author>
    <functionCode code='…' codeSystem='…'
        codeSystemName='…' displayName='…'/>
    <time value='…'/>
    <assignedAuthor>
        <id root='…' extension='…'/>
        <code code='…' codeSystem='…'
            codeSystemName='…' displayName='…'/>
        <addr>…</addr>
        <telecom value='…'/>
        <assignedPerson>
            <name>…</name>
        </assignedPerson>
    </assignedAuthor>
    <representedOrganization>…</representedOrganization>
</author>
```

Fig. 14.25 Author example with a person author

The Data Enterer

The data enterer role is the second of three different kinds of information sources. This is a person who enters the information into the clinical document by transferring it into an information system from other sources, paper forms, transcription of audio, etc. The data enterer does not create new information; they simply transfer it from one medium to

```
<author>
    <functionCode code='…' codeSystem='…'
        codeSystemName='…' displayName='…'/>
    <time value='…'/>
    <assignedAuthor>
        <id root='…' extension='…'/>
        <code code='…' codeSystem='…'
            codeSystemName='…' displayName='…'/>
        <addr>…</addr>
        <telecom value='…'/>
        <assignedAuthoringDevice>
            <code code='…' codeSystem='…'
                codeSystemName='…' displayName='…'/>
            <manufacturerModelName>…</manufacturerModelName>
            <softwareName>…</softwareName>
        </assignedPerson>
    </assignedAuthor>
    <representedOrganization>…</representedOrganization>
</author>
```

Fig. 14.26 Author example with a device author

another. According to the CDA Release 2.0 standard, the purpose for reporting this participant is to support quality control.

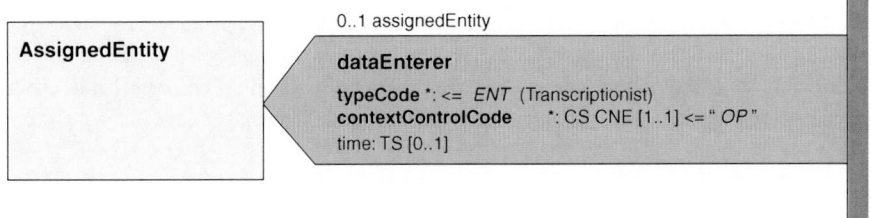

Fig. 14.27 dataEnterer association and AssignedEntity class

The time class attribute captures the starting time of the data enterer's participation.

The AssignedEntity Role

The dataEnterer association class creates a link between the clinical document and the
person assigned to enter the data. If you compare the assignedEntity class above to the
assignedAuthor class used for author you will note only one difference. The player of
role of an assignedEntity class can only be an assignedPerson, whereas for the
assignedAuthor, the player of the role could either be an author or a device. This small
variation between the two is the reason why they are different classes with different names.

The example below shows the XML that can be used to represent a data enterer in a CDA document.

```
<dataEnterer>
    <time value='…/>
    <assignedEntity>
        <id root='…' extension='…'/>
        <code code='…' codeSystem='…'
            codeSystemName='…' displayName='…'/>
        <addr>…</addr>
        <telecom value='…'/>
        <assignedPerson>
            <name>…</name>
        </assignedPerson>
        <representedOrganization>…</representedOrganization>
    </assignedEntity>
</dataEnterer>
```

Fig. 14.28 Data enterer XML example

Information Providers

Information providers are the third kind of information source for a CDA document. These are people who provide information about the patient, and may include patients themselves, parents or guardians, other care givers, or even simply someone who witnessed the events that occurred to the patient. The informant association class links the CDA document to the people that provide information about the patient.

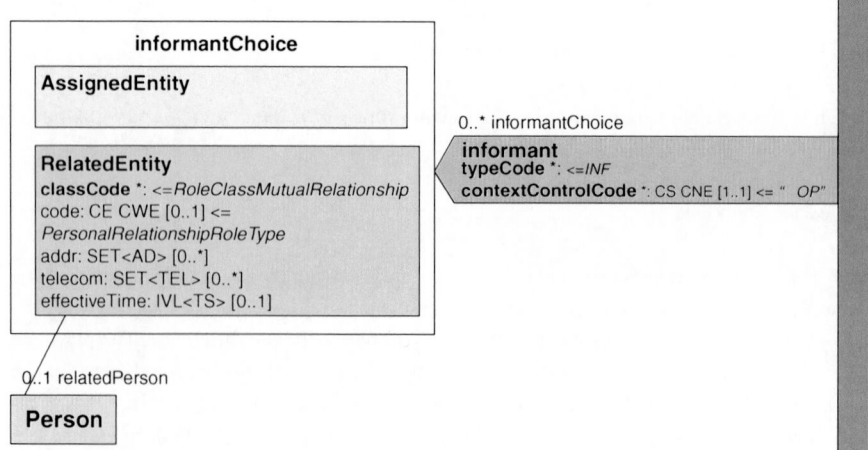

Fig. 14.29 informance association and relatedEntity classes

The main purpose is to capture the identity of the person providing the information, and their relationship to the patient, for follow-up or evaluation of the information provided, so the participation `time` does not appear in the model.

The `assignedEntity` class can be used when the person providing the information is another healthcare provider or employee of the organization providing care. For example, a nurse reporting on the patient condition or response to medication could be an informant.

The `relatedEntity` class is used when the person providing the information has some defined relationship to the patient. These relationships could be formal, as in the relationships between a patient and their legally authorized agent (e.g., a healthcare proxy), or informal as in a caregiver, family member or friend.

The `classCode` of the `relatedEntity` class further refines the type of relationship using values in the `RoleClassMutualRelationship` value set of the HL7 `RoleClass` vocabulary. The most common code used in the `relatedEntity` class in CDA instances is PRS, which represents a person with personal relationship (usually a familial one) with the patient. This code would commonly be used in pediatric care where an infant's mother or father reports signs and symptoms, or in inpatient care where a family member reports what happened to a patient. In these cases the `code` class attribute further specifies the kind of relationship, and would usually come from the HL7 `PersonalRelationshipRole` type value set of the HL7 `RoleCode` vocabulary.

When the related entity is not a person in a personal relationship with the patient, other value sets are more appropriate for the `code` class attribute.

The example below shows how an informant would be represented in XML in a CDA document.

```
<informant typeCode="INF">
   <relatedEntity classCode="PRS">
      <code code='...' codeSystem='...'
         codeSystemName='...' displayName='...'/>
      <addr>...</addr>
      <telecom value='...'/>
      <effectiveTime value='...'/>
      <relatedPerson>
         <name>...</name>
      </relatedPerson>
   </relatedEntity>
</informant>
```

Fig. 14.30 Informant XML example

Co-occurrence

A feature of `role` classes is that the `classCode` class attribute represents a large grained classification of the type of role. That often suggests a value set to further specify the role details in the `code` attribute of the `role` class. This dependence of the `code` attribute on the `classCode` attribute represents a *co-occurrence* constraint. Co-occurrence constraints are not easily transformed into W3C Schema rules. Co-occurrence constraints are discussed in more detail in the chapter on Templates starting on page 263.

The Steward

Every valid CDA document must have a steward according to the standard. The steward is the organization that is responsible for maintaining a true and accurate copy of the document for as long as is required by local policy. The steward is associated with the clinical document through the custodian participation class.

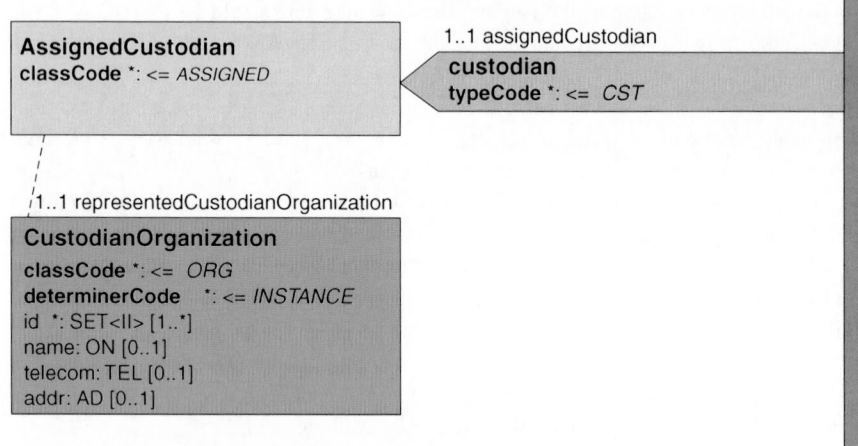

Fig. 14.31 custodian association and AssignedCustodian classes

The custodian association links the assigned custodian to the clinical document. The assigned custodian is the organization that has been assigned the role to be the steward of the clinical document.

```
<custodian>
   <assignedCustodian>
      <representedCustodianOrganization>
         <id root='…' extension='…'/>
         <name>…</name>
         <telecom value='…'/>
         <addr>…</addr>
      </representedCustodianOrganization>
   </assignedCustodian>
</custodian>
```

Fig. 14.32 Custodian example

Recipients

Just as there are information sources, there are also recipients of the information. These are associated with the clinical document through the informationRecipient association class.

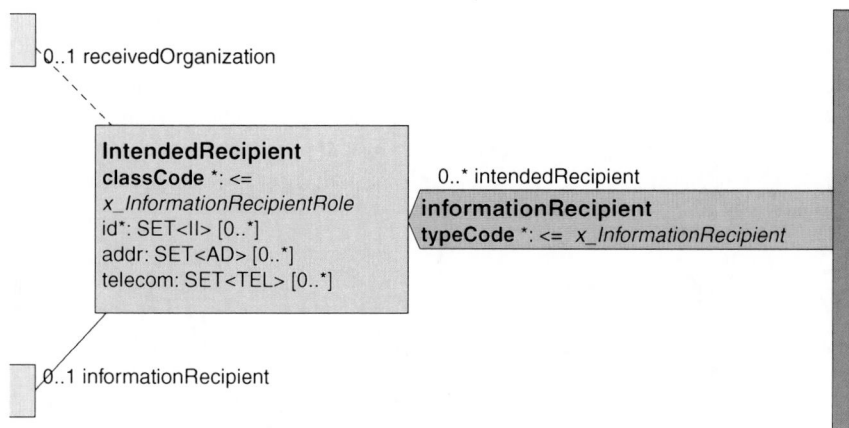

Fig. 14.33 informationRecipient association and intendedRecipient classes

The informationRecipient participation does not include a time class attribute because the time of this person's participation cannot be predicted in advance. The intended recipient can be either an assigned entity, or the health chart associated with an organization. In actual practice, this most often uses the assigned entity class code (ASSIGNED).

The player for this role is also named informationRecipient in the CDA model (and in the XML). The recievedOrganization scopes the role, and usually represents the organization that employs the informationRecipient.

```
<informationRecipient>
   <intendedRecipient classCode="ASSIGNED">
       <id root='…' extension='…'/>
       <addr>…</addr>
       <telecom value='…'/>
       <informationRecipient>
           <name>…</name>
       </informationRecipient>
       <receivedOrganization>…</receivedOrganization>
   </intendedRecipient>
</informationRecipient>
```

Fig. 14.34 Information Recipient XML example

Signers of the Document

One of the key properties of the CDA document is the potential for authentication. This is in some ways like "persuit of happiness" enumerated as one of the unalienable rights in the US Constitution. Just because the potential exists does not mean that every clinical document will be signed.

There are two different types of authenticators that can sign a CDA document. An authenticator simply attests by their signature that the information in the document is true and correct to the best of their knowledge. The legal authenticator's signature however, conveys that the person signing the document takes legal responsibility for its content.

In CDA, organizations do not take legal responsibility, only individuals can do so on behalf of an organization. Also, the legal authenticator takes responsibility for the entire content of the clinical document. There is no way to sign just part of one.

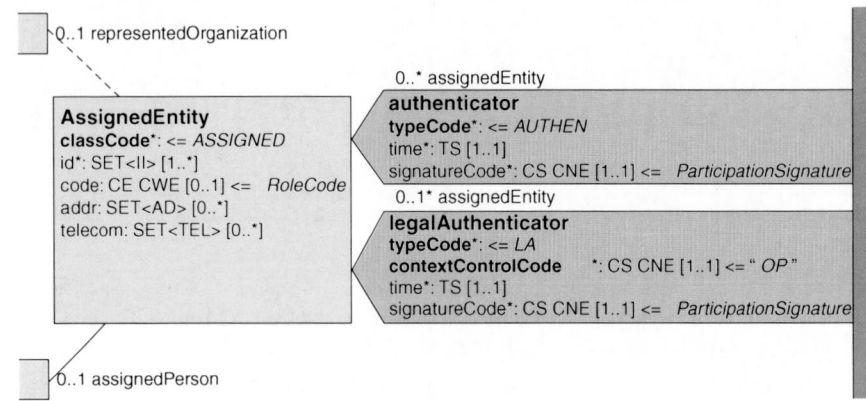

Fig. 14.35 authenticator and legalAuthenticator association and AssignedEntity classes

The time of signing is captured in the `time` class attribute of the `authenticator` and `legalAuthenticator` class. The `signatureCode` attribute carries a code of S to indicate that their *electronic signature* has been attached. Two other code values are permitted, a code of X indicates that this participants signature is required (but has not been attached), and a code of I indicates that the participant intends to sign the document. Appearance of either of these two code values indicates that the document has not been signed by the participant. Only the value S is commonly seen, because when the document has not been signed, the `authenticator` or `legalAuthenticator` associations are typically not transmitted.

The X and I codes support document signing workflows, but this metadata is normally not carried in the CDA content. Instead it is managed through the workflow application. These class attributes can be used by applications to save intermediate (non-final) content in CDA form, and maintain the appropriate signature status.

These associations use the `assignedEntity` role to identify the person signing the document.

Applications sometimes use CDA extension to include the *digital signature* in the CDA document. This extension adds a `signatureText` element after the `signatureCode` element in the XML representation to carry an XML Advanced Electronic Digital Signature.

Participation signatures attest to a specific action performed by the signer. In the case of the authenticator signature, the most common use case is for the author to attest that this is in fact the text they produced. You might ask why that signature is not then attached to the author, especially if you have never encountered a transcription workflow. In many healthcare facilities, clinical documents are created by transcription of an audio recording, and it is only after the transcribed text is reviewed by the author that the document is signed. In these cases, the original author of the content is not always available to sign the content. Local policies often allow for supervising physicians to sign for physicians who are not available to sign a clinical document. Separating the authenticator and legal authenticator participations for the purpose of signing the document from the author allows these workflows to be completed and still record both the signer and the author of the content separately.

The example below shows how an authenticator or legal authenticator would be represented in the XML of a CDA document. The XML for the assigned entity can be found in Fig. 14.28 above.

```
<legalAuthenticator> <!-- OR --> <authenticator>
    <time value='…'/>
    <signatureCode code="S"/>
    <assignedEntity>…</assignedEntity>
</legalAuthenticator> <!-- OR --> </authenticator>
```

Fig. 14.36 Authenticator and legal authenticator XML example

Other Participants

The last participant supported in the CDA document is a generic one. This participant allows CDA to record associate other roles with a clinical document to support use cases not originally anticipated.

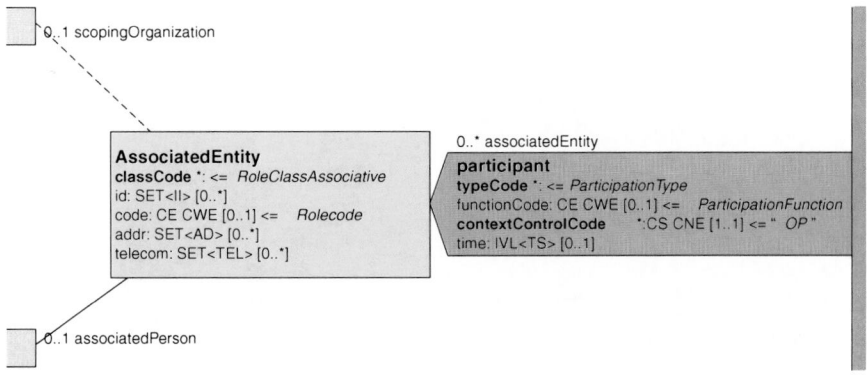

Fig. 14.37 participation association and associatedEntity classes

The participant association class allows the functionCode to be recorded to identify the *functional role* of the participant. It is also the only participation in the CDA header that allows the time of participation to be recorded using an interval of time (IVL_TS).

The generic participation class uses the associated entity role. This is a very generic role which basically can capture the association of two entities. However, CDA also restricts this association to be between a person (found in the `associatedPerson` class), and an organization (found in the `scopingOrganization` class).

The presence of the generic `participation` class in CDA results in multiple representations of a CDA document that could be semantically equivalent. One could use this `participation` to record an author, and the content would be semantically correct according to the RIM. However the CDA standard has this to say about the class in section 4.2.2.9: The participant is "Used to represent other participants not explicitly mentioned by other classes…"

This prohibits used of the `participant` class to represent any class already represented in the CDA model. This is also common usage in CDA implementations. Some implementations have used the more expansive capabilities (e.g., with respect to `functionCode` and time) of the `participant` class to augment the clinical document content with more than is allowed in the intended classes. This is not harmful when the class intended to represent the information is also present and duplicates information in other participations. That is because CDA implementations do not commonly look in the `participant` class for participations already specified elsewhere in the standard.

```
<participant typeCode="IND">
   <functionCode code='…' codeSystem='…'
      codeSystemName='…' displayName='…'/>
   <time value='…'/>
   <associatedEntity classCode="NOK">
      <id root='…' extension='…'/>
      <code code="MTH"
         codeSystem="2.16.840.1.113883.5.111"
         codeSystemName="RoleCode" displayName="Mother"/>
      <addr>…</addr>
      <telecom value='…'/>
      <associatedPerson>
         <name>…</name>
      </associatedPerson>
      <scopingOrganization>…</scopingOrganization>
   </associatedEntity>
</participant>
```

Fig. 14.38 Participant XML example

14.4
People, Organizations and Devices

These classes represent the various entities or "nouns" used in the clinical statements. They may be the subject of the document (such as the patient), or creators, providers, maintainers or recipients of the information in the clinical document.

Patient

The patient class describes the person who is the patient in the context of the clinical document and appears in the figure on the following page. *In CDA Release 2, the patient is also implicitly the subject of the information found in the clinical document.* As a result, a number of details about the patient are captured in class attributes on the patient class. These class attributes capture important social, clinical and administrative information about the patient.

Identifiers

The id class attribute on the patient class was carried forward from CDA Release 1 to CDA Release 2. It was meant in CDA Release 1 to capture a single unique identifier for the person.

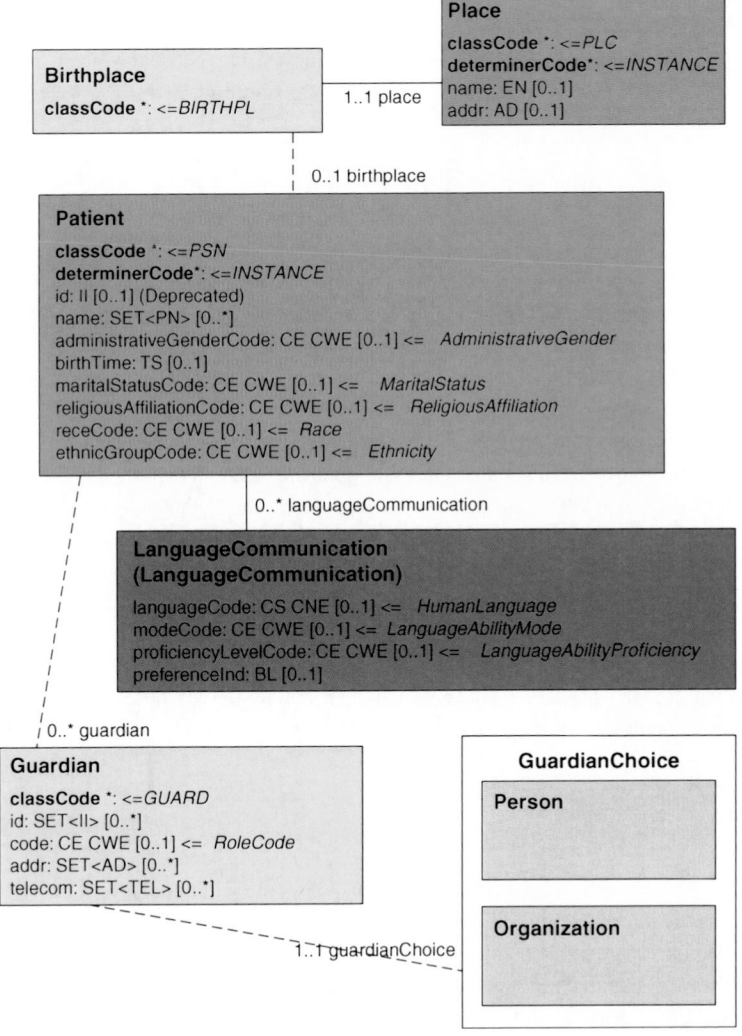

Fig. 14.39 The patient class

The id class attribute was deprecated in CDA Release 2 because there really is no single identifier for a person. There may be a number of other identifiers for a patient, but these are associated with the patient through roles. For example, the patient may be identified as a citizen of a country, a driver in a locale, a member of an organization, etc. But these identifiers belong on a role class associated with the patient.

The attribute is sometimes used sometimes in current implementations to store the identifier for the patient as might be stored in a master patient index.

Names

The name class attribute can appear any number of times in the patient class to capture the various names by which the patient may be known. These names include their current legal name, the name by which they might wish to be called, names used in the past, etc.

Table 7.1 on page 67 and Table 7.2 on page 68 describe how to identify different types of names, and their uses respectively. The Entity Name data type from which Person Name is derived from allows these names to indicate the time in which they were used (see <validTime> on page 69).

Gender

The administrativeGenderCode class attribute describes the gender of the patient used for administrative, rather than clinical purposes. The concept of gender for administrative purposes is much simpler than the same concept as used clinically. Clinically the concept of gender may need to address not just genetic, but also expressed, anatomical, and hormonal gender.

This class attribute recommends the use of the HL7 AdministrativeGender codes. These codes include three different values to describe gender as male, female, and undifferentiated. The latter case is one where the gender is not unknown, rather the patient does not express gender in a way that they could be differentiated between male and female. The administrativeGenderCode class attribute can also be transmitted as being unknown, as might be the case in emergency situations where the patient has yet to be identified. In these cases, the class attribute is transmitted using a flavor of null (see nullFlavor on page 35).

Other vocabularies may be used to transmit administrative gender. Some local policies require the use of a particular vocabulary, which is why the HL7 AdministrativeGender vocabulary is only recommended, not required.

Marital Status

The maritalStatusCode class attribute captures the patient's current marital status. Marital status may have policy implications regarding who may see the patient or how clinical decisions are made regarding their treatment when the patient is unable to participate in that decision making process. It also may also help to identify the type of follow up care needed for a patient who may require assistance following treatment.

Religion

The `religiousAffiliationCode` class attribute captures the affiliation of the patient with a particular religion. In some locales, policy prohibits this information from being stored in the medical record, and others allow it. Availability of this information allows healthcare facilities to provide care for the patient in a way that shows respect to their religious beliefs.

Race and Ethnicity

The `raceCode` and `ethnicGroupCode` class attributes allow information about the patient racial and ethnic affiliations to be expressed. Race and ethnicity information may be used to help assess the risk of a patient with respect to particular conditions. In some locales (e.g., the US) this information may also be used operationally to detect racial and ethnic disparities in the way patients are treated. In others, transmission of this information in a medical record is prohibited.

Language

The `languageCommunication` class allows the patient's language capability and preferences to be expressed. This class appears in HL7 diagrams in blue because it falls outside of the backbone, have none of properties of an act, participation, role or entity.

The `languageCode` class attribute represents the language which the patient has some ability. The `modeCode` class attribute indicates whether this ability is spoken, written, read or signed.

The `proficiencyLevelCode` class attribute can be used to provide an assessment of the patient's ability with this language.

Finally the `preferenceInd` class attribute indicates which language or languages the patient prefers to communicate in.

Birth Place

The patient's birth place is recorded as a role association between the patient class and a place of birth. The `birthplace` association class links the `patient` class together with the `place` class. The `patient` scopes the role played by place in this association.

See places below for more detail on the `place` class.

Guardians

A patient may have one or more guardians who are responsible for the care of the patient. The role of guardian may be played by either a person or an organization (see the `person` and `organization` entity classes below for details).

The id class attribute on the guardian is used to identify the guardian person or organization in that role. The code class attribute can be used to further specify the type of guardianship.

Places

The place class represents a place that may be recorded as a location of care, or the place of birth of a patient. The place can have either a name or address or both. These are found in the name and addr class attributes respectively.

The example below show the XML used to represent the patient.

```
<patient>
   <name>…</name>
   <administrativeGenderCode code='…' displayName='…'
      codeSystem='…' codeSystemName='…'/>
   <birthTime value='…'/>
   <maritalStatusCode code='…' displayName='…'
      codeSystem='…' codeSystemName='…'/>
   <religiousAffiliationCode code='…' displayName='…'
      codeSystem='…' codeSystemName='…'/>
   <raceCode code='…' displayName='…'
      codeSystem='…' codeSystemName='…'/>
   <ethnicGroupCode code='…' displayName='…'
      codeSystem='…' codeSystemName='…'/>
   <birthplace>
      <place><name>…</name><addr>…</addr></place>
   </birthplace>
   <guardian>
      <code code='…' displayName='…'
         codeSystem='' codeSystemName='RoleCode'/>
      <!-- One of the following two elements -->
      <guardianPerson><name>…</name></guardianPerson>
      <guardianOrganization>…</guardianOrganization>
   </guardian>
</patient>
```

Fig. 14.40 patient XML example

Organizations

Organizations are used in many places in the CDA model. Assigned roles such as author, authenticator, or recipient represent an organization, products are manufactured by an organization, healthcare facilities are run by service provider organizations, etc. All of these organizations use the same class structure.

Organizations can be identified using the id class attribute. They may be known by multiple names which are found in the name class attribute. The standardIndustryClass-Code can be used to identify the type of organization using an industry classification system.

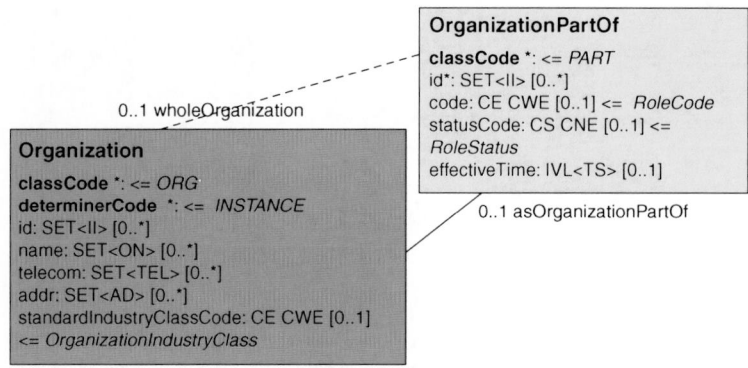

Fig. 14.41 Organization and OrganizationPartOf classes

organizations are often hierarchically structured. The `OrganizationPartOf` association class allows one to walk up the organizational structure.

These class attributes are sufficient when the organization is simply associated with an assigned or other role, because the person associated with the role is the focus of the association.

The XML used to represent an organization appears in the figure below. This example shows a guardian organization that is part of a larger organization, repeating itself in the `<wholeOrganization>` element.

```
<guardianOrganization>
    <id root='…' extension='…'/>
    <name>…</name>
    <telecom value='…'/>
    <addr>…</addr>
    <standardIndustryClassCode code='…' displayName='…'
        codeSystem='…' codeSystemName='…'/>
    <asOrganizationPartOf>
        <wholeOrganization>…</wholeOrganization>
    </asOrganizationPartOf>
</guardianOrganization>
```

Fig. 14.42 Organization XML example

The only place that uses a different class structure for an organization in CDA release 2 is in the custodian. Representation of the organization acting as a steward (or custodian) of a clinical document has additional requirements. It is the organization rather than a person that is the focus of the custodial participation. The principal of stewardship means that you should be able to locate the organization that maintains the true and accurate original of the clinical document.

You may have noted that the id class attribute of the `custodianOrganization` class is required whereas in the `organization` class it is optional. While organizations may be known by several names, and have several addresses and phone numbers, only one each of

Fig. 14.43 The CustodianOrganization class

CustodianOrganization

classCode *: <= *ORG*
determinerCode *: <= *INSTANCE*
id *: SET<II> [1..*]
name: ON [0..1]
telecom: TEL [0..1]
addr: AD [0..1]

---

the name, addr and telecom class attributes is provided for the custodianOrganization class. These class attributes should be filled with the best information one would
want to have to locate an original document.

The XML used to represent the custodian organization is shown in the example below.

```
<custodianOrganization>
   <id root='…' extension='…'/>
   <name>…</name>
   <telecom value='…'/>
   <addr>…</addr>
</custodianOrganization>
```

Fig. 14.44 CustodianOrganization example

Persons

The person class is used to carry the name of different people assigned or playing the
various roles in the clinical document. In the clinical document header, only the patient
receives special attention. All other cases focus principally upon the role of the person,
rather than their personal attributes. The name class attribute is the only additional information supplied by this class.

Fig. 14.45 The person class

Person

classCode *: <= *PSN*
determinerCode *: <= *INSTANCE*
name: SET<PN> [0..*]

Sample XML used to represent the person is shown in the figure below. *Because the
<name> element uses a mixed content model, white space is added for readability inside
the element delimiters, instead of in the text content. This is an old trick well known by
SGML markup language enthusiasts.*

```
<person>
   <name><prefix>…</prefix
      ><given>…</given
      ><given>…</given
      ><family>…</family
      ><suffix>…</suffix
   ></name>
</person>
```

Fig. 14.46 Person XML example

Devices

While most clinical documents will be created principally by a person with the help of a computer system, some may be created almost wholly by a computer system. In these cases, it is reasonable to capture information about this system and the person responsible for maintaining it. This is done through the `authoringDevice` class shown below.

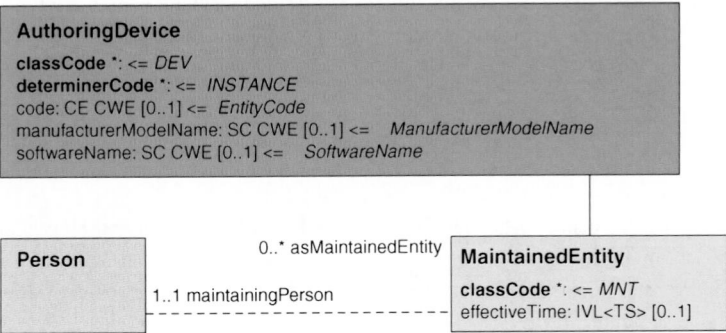

Fig. 14.47 The AuthoringDevice and MaintainingEntity classes

The `code` class attribute allows the type device to be described. The `manufacturerModelName` and `softwareName` allow different components of the device to be described. A device may be maintained by a number of individuals, each of which may also be associated with the device through the `maintainedEntity` role.

The example below shows the XML used for an authoring device.

```
<assignedAuthoringDevice>
    <code …/>
    <manufacturerModelName>...</manufacturerModelName>
    <softwareName>…</softwareName>
</assignedAuthoringDevice>
```

Fig. 14.48 assignedAuthoringDevice XML example

Summary

- The CDA Header sets the context for the clinical document.
- The XML appears in the order of class attributes, participant associations and then act associations.
- Class attributes in the `ClinicalDocument` class identify the document, describe what is in it, indicate relevant dates and aid in securing the content.
- Every clinical document has a single unique identity that it is known by and that identity is recorded in it.

- LOINC® is the preferred vocabulary for classifying documents.
- The CDA document header requires at least one author and patient, and one and only one custodian (steward).
- Other information producers described in the CDA header include the transcriptionist (data enterer) and the informant.
- The CDA document header can also record signers of the document, intended recipients, and a wide variety of other participants as needed.
- The CDA header can describe encounters, services, documents which are replaced or added to, orders that it fulfills, and consents that were obtained.

Questions

1. Create a CDA document header containing only mandatory content. How many elements are in the XML?
2. Create a CDA document containing only required or mandatory content. How many elements are in the XML?
3. Which participation associations are required to be present in the `ClinicalDocument` class?
4. CDA documents require a number of different identifiers, for example, for the patient, encounter, associated providers, etc. How many different kinds of identifiers are mandatory?
5. How many different kinds of identifiers are required?
6. In what ways does the `ServiceEvent` class differ from other clinical statements found elsewhere in the body of the clinical document?

Research Questions

1. What coding systems are preferred in your region to describe the classes found in the CDA header in more detail?
2. What organizations are responsible for maintaining these code systems and how would you provide feedback on their content?
3. What are the local policies in your region regarding capture and transmission of religion, race and ethnicity data? Is this practice required, promoted, discouraged or prohibited?

References

1. RFC 3066, Tags for the Identification of Languages, January 2001, Internet Engineering Task Force. Available on the web at http://www.ietf.org/rfc/rfc3066.txt

2. Codes for the Representation of Names of Languages, United States Library of Congress, Available on the web at http://www.loc.gov/standards/iso639-2/php/code_list.php
3. English Country Names and Code Elements, ISO, Available on the web at http://www.iso.org/iso/country_codes/iso_3166_code_lists/english_country_names_and_code_elements.htm
4. Latanya Sweeney, Uniqueness of Simple Demographics in the U.S. Population, LIDAP-WP4 Carnegie Mellon University, Laboratory for International Data Privacy, 20001Xxxx

The CDA body represents the narrative content of the clinical document. The body is simply a part of the clinical document, and is accessed through the component association class.

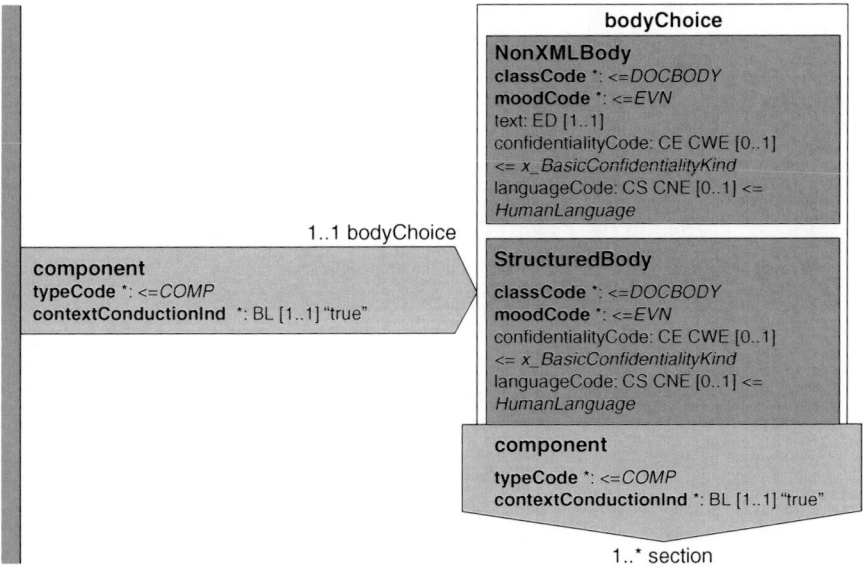

Fig. 15.1 The CDA body

There are two choices for the body content. It can be stored in an unstructured format using the NonXMLBody class. It can also be structured using the structuredBody class.

The class attributes of these two acts are nearly identical. The confidentialityCode class attribute serves essentially the same purpose as the class attribute of the same name on the ClinicalDocument. The only difference is that it identifies the sensitivity of the content found in (or below) the body of the document, and does not address sensitivity of information found in the document header. Since the sensitivity of the clinical document is at least as sensitive as its most sensitive component, this class attribute is rarely used.

K.W. Boone, *The CDA™ Book*,
DOI: 10.1007/978-0-85729-336-7_15, © Springer-Verlag London Limited 2011

The languageCode class attribute identifies the primary human language used in the narrative content. Again, this duplicates the attribute found in the ClinicalDocument class and so is also rarely used.

The difference between these two classes is in how they communicate the narrative content. The NonXMLBody class communicates the content in the text class attribute. The StructuredBody class communicates the content using the section classes associated with the StructuredBody though additional component association classes.

15.1
Unstructured Narrative

The NonXMLBody class communicates the narrative content through the text class attribute. A Level 1 CDA document would use the NonXMLBody class to send the text.

The text class attribute uses the ED (Encapsulated Data) data type, which means that it can effectively carry any binary content, and it can do so by including that content directly in any text format, or be encoded using a base 64 encoded string, or by reference to an external resource.

The example below shows how plain text content can be included in a CDA document. The use of the < ! [CDATA [and]] > delimiters tell the XML parser to ignore any special characters in the content. This allows the plain text to contain ampersands, less than and greater than signs without concern for escaping the content.

```
<component>
 <nonXMLBody>
   <text mediaType='text/plain'><![CDATA[
This is a narrative text report.
]]></text>
 </nonXMLBody>
</component>
```

Fig. 15.2 nonXMLBody example with text content

The same sort of XML could also be used to contain text from other formats such as RTF or HTML.

The next example shows how content from a binary data format such as Portable Document Format (PDF) could be included inside the CDA document. The binary data is simply base 64 encoded (see the discussion of base 64 encoding on page 50) and the resulting string is stored in the <text> element as shown in the figure below.

```
<component>
 <nonXMLBody>
  <text mediaType='application/pdf' representation='B64'>
      JVBERi0xLjMKJcfsj6IKOCAwIG9iago8
      PC9MZW5ndGggOSAwIFIvRmlsdGVyIC9G
         ...
      eHJlZgo0OTkzNAo1JUVPRgo=
  </text>
 </nonXMLBody>
</component>
```

Fig. 15.3 nonXMLBody example with base 64 encoded content

Compression can also be applied to the data contained in this block (before the base 64 encoding is done) to reduce the space that it takes up in the XML representation.

Finally, the text can simply be referenced by a URL. In the example below, a relative URL identifies the file sample.pdf which is co-located with the CDA document.

```
<component>
 <nonXMLBody>
  <text mediaType='application/pdf'><
      reference value='sample.pdf' /></text>
 </nonXMLBody>
</component>
```

Fig. 15.4 nonXMLBody example with referenced content

Separating the narrative content from the CDA document defeats one of the purposes of the CDA standard, but has some benefits. CDA Documents using the nonXMLBody are more difficult to render because the embedded content has to be decompressed, decoded, and handed off to a separate rendering component (e.g., a word processor or viewer application). These operations are more difficult to accomplish than simple transformations of the content that can be viewed in a web browser.

Being able to separate the content can make these operations easier to perform, at the cost of separating the content from the document.

One mechanism that is suggested by the CDA standard uses a MIME multipart package, which serves the function of keeping all of the components together. Section 3 of the CDA standard describes how a CDA document can be sent in a MIME multipart package. The auxiliary files are included in that package and include a content-location header in the MIME part that gives the "filename" that is used to reference the content in the CDA document.

NonXMLBody Means No XML

The NonXMLBody class has that name because the CDA Standard further imposes the constraint that the content will not be in XML. The CDA standard states [§4.3.1.1]: "The NonXMLBody class represents a document body that is in some format other than XML." This constraint was imposed because it was felt that if you had an XML document, it could be restructured into the CDA StructuredBody class via an XSL transform and there was no need to allow for arbitrary XML content.

Some have noted (including this author) that while document based XML formats might be readily converted into the CDA Narrative block format, graphic based formats using XML would not be so easily converted. It also completely fails to address HTML which could be easily transformed, but is not an XML format (it uses the older SGML standard). Under this constraint, a rendering of an ECG report using the Scalable Vector Graphics (SVG) standard is not allowed according to the standard. Simply changing the file format from SVG to SVGZ (compressed SVG) makes the result a binary file, and would seem to meet the requirements of the content being non-XML.

It might be better to state that the content of the text class attribute of the NonXMLBody must appear using something other than the text/xml MIME type. This would allow use of SVG (which has a MIME type of image/svg+xml) in the CDA document, but would prohibit other forms of XML which address text content.

15.2
Structured Narrative

One of the key benefits of the CDA standard is that it can make applications less prone to failure due to proprietary file formats. The use of a standard format for narrative content makes it possible to faithfully reproduce the text decades after it has been stored. The structuredBody class is the starting point for this content. This class is simply composed of (using component associations) a number of different section class instances.

```
<component>
   <structuredBody>
      <!-- one or more sections -->
      <component>
         <section>…</section>
      </component>
   </structuredBody>
</component>
```

Fig. 15.5 structuredBody XML example

Section

The section class contains information for one part of the CDA document. The model for the section class is shown in the figure below.

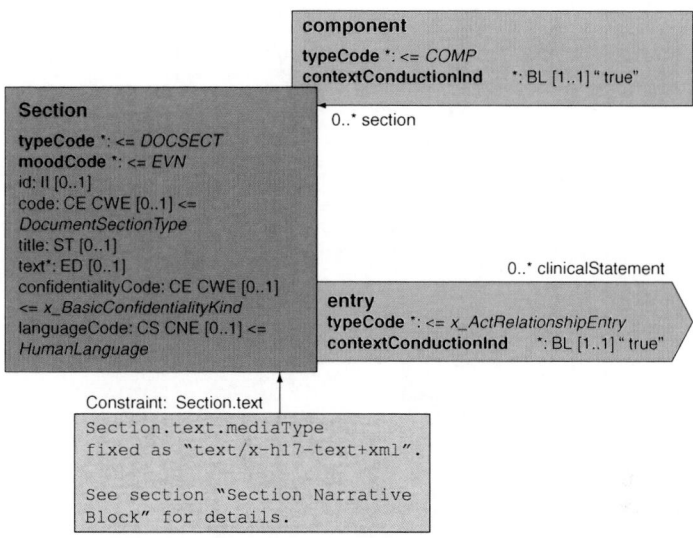

Fig. 15.6 The section class

Each section can be uniquely identified using the `id` class attribute. Use of this attribute allows the entire section to be referenced in other content.

The `code` class attribute classifies the section for machine processing. It serves similar purposes for computer processing as the `title` class attribute does for human use. It allows the content of the section to be quickly classified. The CDA standard prefers the use of LOINC for the content of the `code` class attribute, but other vocabularies are permitted, and are even required in some regions. The distinction between a level 1 and level 2 CDA is that the latter uses both the `structuredBody` class and the `code` class attribute for each section. The example below shows the XML used for a narrative section.

```
<component>
   <section>
      <id root='…' extension='…'/>
      <code code='…' displayName='…'
         codeSystem='2.16.1.113883.6.1'
         codeSystemName='LOINC' />
      <title>…</title>
      <text>…</text>
      <subject>…</subject>
      <author>…</author>
      <informant>…</informant>
      <!-- See Clinical Statements -->
      <entry>…</entry>
      <!-- Optional subsections -->
      <component><section>…</section></component>
   </section>
</component>
```

Fig. 15.7 CDA section XML

The section class contains two human readable class attributes, title and text. Both are meant to be rendered for human readability. The following XSLT fragment can be used to render a <section> element.

```
<!-- Render a CDA Section -->
<xsl:template match='cda:section'>
   <!-- Compute a section number to create an ID -->
   <xsl:variable name='secnum'>
       <xsl:number level='any' count='cda:section'/>
   </xsl:variable>
   <!-- generate each subsection in a division -->
   <div class='section'>
       <!-- render the section title -->
       <div class='title' id='_section-{$secnum}'>
           <xsl:value-of select='cda:title'/>
       </div>
       <div id='_body-section-{$secnum}'>
           <!-- render the section content -->
           <xsl:apply-templates select='cda:text'/>
           <!-- render the sub-sections -->
           <xsl:apply-templates
               select='cda:component/cda:section'/>
       </div>
   </div>
</xsl:template>
<!-- render the narrative text of a section by
     Rendering the elements it contains -->
<xsl:template match='cda:section/cda:text'>
   <xsl:apply-templates select='*|text()'/>
</xsl:template>
```

Fig. 15.8 Rendering a section

The title class attribute provides the human readable heading for the section. This should be the section heading that the provider would normally expect to see as part of their clinical practice. The separation of the title class attribute from code class attribute seems to be duplicative, especially since the code class attribute contains a display name that could be used to describe the section. However, the separation makes sense from a different perspective. Healthcare providers are trained to work a certain way, and imposing arbitrary changes in their work habits is disruptive. The title class attribute can be used to carry the heading for the section that they are accustomed to, while the code class attribute contains what is needed for computer processing. This avoids the situation of making the provider do something different to make it easier for the computer to process the content.

The text class attribute is restricted by the CDA standard to contain content using only the CDA Narrative block format. This format is discussed in more detail in the following section on the Narrative Block.

The confidentialityCode and languageCode class attributes classify the contents of the sections by the level of sensitivity of the data and the primary language that is used, just as for the ClinicalDocument and structuredBody classes. As for the structuredBody class, these class attributes are also infrequently used in implementation.

Sections can be nested. A subsection is connected to its parent section by the component association class. A section can contain both text and subsections but this is not common. When rendering sections containing both text and subsections, the text should appear before subsections.

Each section can also contain multiple machine readable entries. These are associated with the section using the entry association class. The contents of these entries are described in the next chapter covering Clinical Statements in the CDA.

Each section of a CDA document can contain information that was created or provided by different participants than the rest of the document. The author and informant association classes can be used to connect the section with these participants. The definitions and representations of these classes are identical to the similarly named classes described in the previous chapter on The CDA Header.

The subject association links the section to an individual other than the patient and is described following the narrative block.

15.3
The Narrative Block

The text class attribute of the section class appears in an XML format that closely approximates HTML or XHTML. The table below shows how the CDA XML elements can be mapped onto XHTML that has similar syntax.

Table 15.1 CDA narrative block to XHTML mapping

CDA content	XHTML
Direct equivalents	
<sub>	<sub>
<sup>	<sup>
Paragraphs and content	
<paragraph>	<p>
<content>	<span>
Links	
<linkHTML>	<a>

(continued)

Table 15.1 (continued)

CDA content	XHTML
Lists	
`<list listType="ordered">`	`<ol>`
`<list listType="unordered">`	`<ul>`
`<item>`	`<li>`
Tables	
`<colgroup>`, `<thead>`, `<tbody>`, `<table>`, `<caption>`, `<col>`, `<tfoot>`, `<th>`, `<td>` and `<tr>`	Identical
`<footnote><footnoteRef>`	Not available
Images	
`<renderMultimedia>`	`<img>`
Common Attributes	
`ID="value"`	`ID="value"`
`styleCode="className"`	`class="className"`

HTML Equivalents

Many CDA elements have the same names as the XHTML counterpart and serve exactly the same purpose. The `<br/>` element inserts a line break into the output. The `<sub>` and `<sup>` elements mark text that should be shown as a subscript or superscript respectively.

These CDA elements can be easily converted into XHTML using a single template in XSLT.

```
<xsl:template match="cda:br|cda:sup|cda:sub">
   <xsl:element name="{local-name()}">
      <xsl:apply-templates select='@ID|@styleCode'/>
      <xsl:copy-of
         select="@*[local-name() != 'ID' and
                    local-name() != 'styleCode']"
      />
      <xsl:apply-templates select="*|text()"/>
   </xsl:element>
</xsl:template>
```

Fig. 15.9 Rendering line breaks, superscripts and subscripts

Paragraphs and Content

The CDA `<paragraph>` and `<content>` elements do the same thing as the `<p>` and `<span>` elements in XHTML respectively.

```
<paragraph>This is a paragraph of text <content
ID='markedSpan'>with a marked span of content</content>
that can be referenced later.</paragraph>
```

Fig. 15.10 An example `<paragraph>`

These can be translated into XHTML by simply changing the name and processing the contents of these tags.

```
<xsl:template match="cda:paragraph">
   <p>
      <xsl:apply-templates select="@*|*|text()"/>
   </p>
</xsl:template>
<xsl:template match='cda:content'>
   <span>
      <xsl:apply-templates select="@*|*|text()"/>
   </span>
</xsl:template>
```

Links

The CDA `<linkHTML>` element has exactly the same function as the `<a>` element in XHTML. Even the attributes work in the same way.

Lists

CDA has a single list element named `<list>` which contains an attribute `listType` using the values `ordered` and `unordered` to distinguish between those two types of lists. List items are contained in an `<item>` element in CDA, as shown in the examples in the figure below.

```
<list listType='unordered'>
   <item ID='allergy-1'>Cephelaxin</item>
   <item ID='allergy-2'>Penicillin</item>
</list>

<list listType='ordered'>
   <item ID='diagnosis-1'>Myocardial Infarction<item>
   <item ID='diagnosis-2'>Hypertension</item>
</list>
```

Fig. 15.11 List XML examples

XHTML uses the <ol> and <ul> elements for these list types respectively, but they both use the <li> element to contain a list item. When the list type is unspecified in the CDA content, then it should be treated as an unordered list. The following XSLT fragment performs the appropriate translation.

```
<xsl:template match="cda:list[@listType='ordered']" >
   <ol><xsl:apply-templates select="@*|*"/></ol>
</xsl:template>
<xsl:template
   match="cda:list[not(@listType) or
                          @listType='unordered']" >
   <ul><xsl:apply-templates select="@*|*"/></ul>
</xsl:template>
<xsl:template match="cda:item">
   <li><xsl:apply-templates select="@*|*|text()"/></li>
</xsl:template>
```

Fig. 15.12 Rendering lists

Footnotes

One of the capabilities found in CDA but not found in XHTML or HTML is the ability to create footnotes. Footnotes are block level elements that leave a mark in one place, and insert the text content in another (at the bottom of a page or end of the document). The <footnote> element in the CDA Narrative Block format contains the text of the footnote, at the location where the footnote reference would be placed. The <footnoteRef> element allows additional references to a prior footnote to be made.

While HTML does layout information to fit into a browser, it doesn't really have the notion of a page of text since browsers have scroll bars. That makes it difficult to put footnotes at the bottom of the "page" in a browser window. It is quite easy, however, to place the content found in the <footnote> element at the end of the document, or the end of the section it appears in. If you accept this limitation, <footnote> and <footnoteRef> elements are not hard to render in XHTML, they just do not have equivalent elements that support them in XHTML.

Rendering footnotes at the end of a section requires modification of the section template given previously. *The XSLT mode feature allows the same content to be processed twice in different ways.* This feature is used to render footnote content in a separate pass of the stylesheet.

```
<xsl:template match='cda:section'>
   … <!-- existing template content -->
   <xsl:apply-templates mode='footnote'
       select='.//cda:footnote'/>
</xsl:template>

<xsl:template match='cda:footnote'>
   <xsl:variable name='footnote-num'>
       <xsl:number level='any' count='cda:footnote'/>
   </xsl:variable>
   <sup>
       <a href='#_footnote-{$footnote-num}'>
           <xsl:value-of select='$footnote-num'/>
       </a>
   </sup>
</xsl:template>

<xsl:template match='cda:footnote' mode='footnote'>
   <!-- Create a footnote number -->
   <xsl:variable name='footnote-num'>
       <xsl:number level='any' count='cda:footnote'/>
   </xsl:variable>

   <p ID='_footnote-{$footnote-num}>
       <sup>
           <!-- Create an identifier if one exists -->
           <xsl:if test='@ID'>
               <xsl:attribute name='ID'>
                   <xsl:value-of select='@ID'/>
               </xsl:attribute>
           </xsl:if>
           <xsl:value-of select='$footnote-num'/>
       </sup>
       <xsl:apply-templates select='*|text()'/>
   </p>
</xsl:template>
```

Fig. 15.13 Rendering footnotes at the end of a section

There are actually two templates responsible for rendering footnote content. The first of these renders the footnote as a superscripted number at the location where it is found. That number is rendered with an internal hyperlink to the later rendering.

The second template is used to render the footnote content. It operates at a different time during the XSLT processing and so is called using a different mode.

Footnote references are only little bit more difficult. First you have to find the original footnote and then compute its footnote number so that you can render the appropriate linking text.

```
<xsl:template match='footnoteRef'>
  <!-- Find the footnote -->
  <xsl:variable name='theFootnote'
     select='//cda:footnote[@ID=current()/@IDREF'/>
  <!-- Compute the footnote number -->
  <xsl:variable name='footnote-num'>
     <xsl:for-each select='$theFootnote'>
        <xsl:number level='any' count='cda:footnote'/>
     </xsl:for-each>
  </xsl:variable>
  <sup>
     <a href='#{@IDREF}'>
        <xsl:value-of select='$footnote-num'/>
     </a>
  </sup>
</xsl:template>
```

Fig. 15.14 Rendering a footnote reference

If you want to the footnotes to appear at the end of the document instead of at the end of the section, simply move the line added to the template for section elements to the template for the ClinicalDocument element.

Tables

The CDA Narrative Block table model is a mild restriction on the XHTML table model. You can safely translate all table elements and attributes to identically named elements and attributes in the output to get the expected rendering results. The following XSLT fragment will perform the appropriate transformation.

```
<xsl:template match="cda:table|cda:colgroup|cda:col|
  cda:tbody|cda:thead|cda:tfoot|cda:tr|cda:th|cda:td">
  <xsl:element name="{local-name()}">
     <xsl:apply-templates select='@ID|@styleCode'/>
     <xsl:copy-of select="@*[local-name() != 'ID' and
                  local-name() != 'styleCode']"
     />
     <xsl:apply-templates select="*|text()"/>
  </xsl:element>
</xsl:template>
```

Fig. 15.15 Copying a CDA table to XHTML in XSLT

Style Codes

CDA adds a `styleCode` attribute to every element. The `styleCode` attribute can be used to convey a set of rendering style suggestions. *These suggestions in the CDA narrative are merely rendering hints. Receiving applications are not required to use these hints, and in some cases it might not be feasible due to limitations of the rendering device.*

However, a great number of applications use XHTML or HTML to render CDA content. In those cases, there is a very simple way to map the CDA `styleCode` attribute into an appropriate rendering. The vocabulary recommended by the CDA standard for `styleCode` can be mapped to style definitions using the Cascading Style Sheets standard that will produce the desired effect. These definitions accompany the `styleCode` definitions given by the CDA standard in the table on the following page. The rendering application then translates the `styleCode` attribute in the CDA into a `classCode` attribute on the appropriate HTML or XHTML element in the transformed output, and defines a set of styles that produce these effects.

This mechanism suggests ways to extend the `styleCode` vocabulary to use additional CSS classes when rendering documents. Simple add a new class to your CSS stylesheet and use that additional `styleCode` attribute.

For even more control, some CSS attributes could be directly controlled. The schemas in the CDA standard define `styleCode` to be a collection of XML name tokens. That means that each `styleCode` value must begin with a letter colon or underscore and can then be followed by other letters, colons, underscores or digits.

Many CSS style attributes have a single value and the name of the attribute and the value can be concatenated together into a single string that meets the requirements for an XML name token. Thus, a `styleCode` of "color:red" could be used directly control the text color. The example also illustrates at least one problem with this approach. It only supports use of `styleCode` values that can fit the XML name token requirements. You could not use a `styleCode` attribute of "color:#ff0000" to accomplish the same thing because the hash mark is not allowed in XML name tokens.

Table 15.2 CSS rendering for CDA style codes

Code	Definition	CSS class definition
Font style (defines font rendering characteristics.)		
Bold	Render with a bold font.	`font-weight: bold`
Underline	Render with an underlines font.	`text-decoration: underline`
Italics	Render italicized.	`font-style: italic`
Emphasis	Render with some type of emphasis.	`font-weight: small-caps`
Table rule style (defines table cell rendering characteristics.)		
Lrule	Render cell with left-sided rule.	`border-left: 1px`
Rrule	Render cell with right-sided rule.	`border-right: 1px`
Toprule	Render cell with rule on top.	`border-top: 1px`

(continued)

Table 15.2 (continued)

Code	Definition	CSS class definition
Botrule	Render cell with rule on bottom.	`border-bottom: 1px`
Ordered list style (defines rendering characteristics for ordered lists.)		
Arabic	List is ordered using Arabic numerals: 1, 2, 3.	`list-style-type: decimal`
LittleRoman	List is ordered using little Roman numerals: i, ii, iii.	`list-style-type: lower-roman`
BigRoman	List is ordered using big Roman numerals: I, II, III.	`list-style-type: upper-roman`
LittleAlpha	List is ordered using little alpha characters: a, b, c.	`list-style-type: lower-alpha`
BigAlpha	List is ordered using big alpha characters: A, B, C.	`list-style-type: upper-alpha`
Unordered list style (defines rendering characteristics for unordered lists.)		
Disc	List bullets are simple solid discs.	`list-style-type: disc`
Circle	List bullets are hollow discs.	`list-style-type: circle`
Square	List bullets are solid squares.	`list-style-type: square`

Contents of this table are drawn from the HL7 Clinical Document Architecture Release 2.0 standard with permission. Columns 1 and 2 come directly from the standard. Column 3 is the author's interpretation

15.4
Subject Participation

The `author` and `informant` association classes in the CDA Body are structured identically to the classes of the same name in the CDA Header. But the `subject` association is a new class. This associates a `section` with a person whose role is recorded in the `relatedSubject` class.

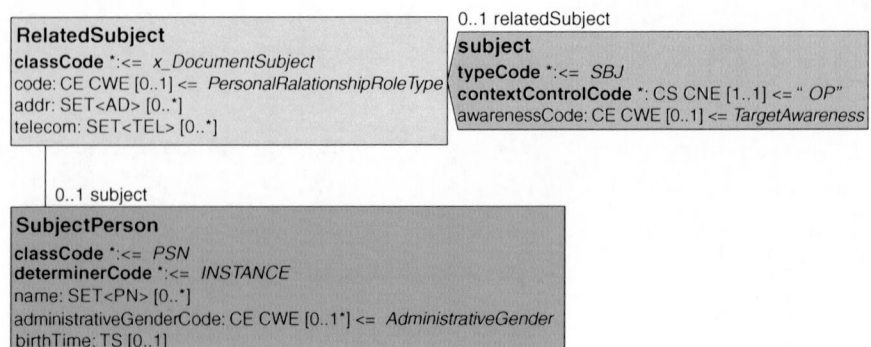

Fig. 15.16 The Subject association and relatedSubject classes

The player of the role is described in the `subjectPerson` class. The `classCode` attribute of this role is limited to two values. When the value is PAT, the subject is another patient, and the scoper is the provider. When the value is PRS, the subject is someone in a personal relationship with the patient, and is scoped by the patient. Since the scoper is already fully defined in the CDA header, it is not separately recorded.

The `subject` participation is typically used in sections which capture family history about a specific family member (the subject). Most often it would be used in labor and delivery settings to record information about the mother in a document for a newborn, or vice versa. In these cases, `classCode` would have the value PRS.

This participation could also be used to show transmission of disease between two patients of the same provider, or for tissue matching, et cetera. In these cases, the `class-Code` would have the value PAT.

The `awarenessCode` class attribute of the `subject` association class indicates whether the person that is the subject of the section is aware of what is stated in its contents. The preferred values for this attribute appear in the table below. This attribute is optional and not often used, but could be important in cases where sensitive information such as disease risk is being recorded. For example, in genetic counseling, risk of disease for a patient is often computed based on risks assessed for other family members for whom the patient has provided a family history. These risks may be recorded in the genetic risk assessment for the patient. It would be important to record whether this information has been communicated to the subject of the assessment since it is very likely to have been made without the awareness of those family members.

Table 15.3 Target awareness

Code	Display name	Description
D	Denying	Target person has been informed about the issue but currently denies it
F	Fully aware	Target person is fully aware of the issue.
I	Incapable	Target person is not capable of comprehending the issue.
M	Marginal	Target person is marginally aware of the issue.
P	Partial	Target person is partially aware of the issue.
U	Uninformed	Target person has not yet been informed of the issue.

Contents of this table are drawn from the HL7 Vocabulary Standard with permission

The `relatedSubject` class indicates the relationship between the `subject` and the `patient` in the code class attribute. Codes for this attribute should be selected from the HL7 PersonalRelationship RoleType value set. The value set contains a great number of family relationships, including first, second and third degree relatives by blood or marriage. It also includes friends, neighbors, roommates and domestic partners. This value set comes from the HL7 RoleCode vocabulary.

The `subjectPerson` class provides some demographic details about the person that is the subject of the section. These details include their name, administrative gender and birth date. These are found in the `name`, `administrativeGender` and `birthTime` class attributes respectively.

The example below shows use of subject to identify one of the natural children born to a mother during the course of a labor and delivery.

```
<section>
   ...
   <subject awarenessCode='I'>
      <relatedSubject classCode='PRS'>
         <code code='NCHILD' displayName='Natural Child'
            codeSystem='2.16.840.1.113883.5.111'
            codeSystemName='RoleCode'/>
         <subject>
            <name>...</name>
            <administrativeGenderCode
               code='F' displayName='Female'
               codeSystem='2.16.840.1.113883.5.1'
               codeSystemName='AdministrativeGender'/>
            <birthTime value='...'/>
         </subject>
      </relatedSubject>
   <subject>
</section>
```

Fig. 15.17 Subject example

15.5
Other Rendering Options

The examples given above for rendering of a CDA document make use of XSLT. There are other options for creating a human readable display of a CDA document. One option is to use a CSS stylesheet with the CDA XML. This works almost in the same way as the XSLT stylesheet. The advantage to using a CSS stylesheet is that it can often be much smaller and simpler that the similarly functioning XSLT stylesheet. However, the CSS standard does not support rearranging content, or displaying information contained in XML attributes.

A third possibility is to render the content using the Formatting Objects defined by the XML Stylesheet Language or XSL. XSLT is a subset of XSL used for transformations. The XSL standard is used to create printed or displayed pages, and includes a wide variety of formatting objects in which this can be done.

Output from systems supporting XSL Formatting Objects is often created using the Portable Document Format. Another way to generate PDF from the CDA output is to use XSLT to convert the CDA to XHTML, and then generate a PDF from the resulting XHTML.

Finally, you can also create Rich Text Formatted output from CDA, also using XSLT. XSLT is not limited to producing XML output. It can also produce HTML or plain text output.

Summary

- The `<nonXMLBody>` element of the CDA document can contain or point to the contents of a file that contains the narrative.
- The `<structuredBody>` element can be used to store an HTML-like representation of the narrative.
- The narrative body is stored in either the `<text>` element of the `<nonXMLBody>` or in `<section>` elements contained in the `<structuredBody>`.
- Both the `<title>` and the `<text>` elements of a `<section>` are meant to be rendered to provide the human readable display.
- The `<code>` element does for a computer what the `<title>` element does for a human.
- Sections can have subsections. The depth of nesting is not limited by the CDA standard.
- The CDA table model is almost identical to the XHTML table model.
- The `<subject>` element associates a CDA `<section>` (and its subsections) with a new subject of discourse other than the patient.

Questions

1. How would you prevent special XML characters from being interpreted in the `<text>` element of a `<nonXMLBody>`?
2. What does the CDA `<component>` XML represent? Why is it present in the CDA model?
3. How would you indicate that information in a particular `<section>` element was provided by a particular person?
4. The CDA `<table>`, `<caption>`, `<col>`, `<colgroup>`, `<thead>`, `<tbody>`, `<tfoot>`, `<th>`, `<td>` and `<tr>` elements are also used as elements in what other standard?
5. There are three other CDA elements that are identically defined in the standard mentioned in the question above. What are they?
6. How would you indicate the formatting for a span of text in a paragraph of CDA content?
7. Who is usually the subject of discourse in the `<text>` in a CDA `<section>`?

Research Questions

1. How would you indicate what has changed between a CDA document and the version that it replaced?
2. What CDA header classes would you use to link a PDF image of a CDA document to its original CDA format? The CDA™ Body

Clinical Statements in the CDA™

16

The CDA contains the original Clinical Statement model used in HL7. The clinical statement model as defined in the CDA standard went on to become a standard of its own in HL7, and is now the foundation of other standards in HL7. As a result, understanding the clinical statement model in CDA can help you understand many other HL7 Version 3 standards.

The clinical statement model includes a number of different act classes to choose from. Each class can be connected to other classes in this model through actRelationship associations. There are a set of participations

16.1
Act Classes in the CDA Clinical Statement Model

There are seven key classes in the clinical statement model: observation, substanceAdministration, supply, procedure, encounter, organizer and act. These appear in XML `<entry>` elements in a CDA `<section>` to record machine readable clinical data. These can be connected to each other using the `<entryRelationship>` element to build larger clinical statements.

The section below describes these classes by starting with the most basic, the act, and building upwards from that to more complex statements. In so doing, it identifies structural similarities of the different classes that are not necessarily reflected in the class hierarchy of the RIM. This is an alternate viewpoint of how the classes work from a software engineering, rather than a clinical information modeling perspective.

act

The `act` class in the RIM is the base class describing all actions for which some record can be made. In the CDA standard, this class is reserved for describing more generic clinical acts for which there is not a more detailed class representation. However, the class attributes found in the `act` class will have the same general meaning in the other classes.

K.W. Boone, *The CDA™ Book*,
DOI: 10.1007/978-0-85729-336-7_16, © Springer-Verlag London Limited 2011

Fig. 16.1 The Act class

> **Act**
>
> **classCode** *: <= x_ActClassDocumentEntryAct
> **moodCode** *: <= x_DocumentActMood
> id: SET<II> [0..*]
> code*: CD CWE [1..1] <= ActCode
> negationInd: BL [0..1]
> text: ED [0..1]
> statusCode: CS CNE [0..1] <= ActStatus
> effectiveTime: IVL<TS> [0..1]
> priorityCode: CE CWE [0..1] <= ActPriority
> languageCode: CS CNE [0..1] <= HumanLanguage

The act class can represent any kind of clinical act. The CDA standard restricts the values of the classCode class attribute to one of the values shown in Table 16.1 below. The act being described can be a proposal (PRP), promise (PRMS), intent (INT) or request (RQO), an appointment (APT) or appointment request (ARQ), a definition (DEF), or the actual occurrence of an event (EVN). These appear in the actMood class attribute.

The identifier of the act appears in the id class attribute. Any act that needs to be tracked through time should have an id associated with it, and so this class attribute should always be valued.

The code class attribute is required by the standard, and further describes the act being performed. There are a few cases where the act is known but the code is not, and so the code class attribute can be filled in using one of the null flavors.

Table 16.1 x_ActClassDocumentEntryAct Values

Code	Display name	Brief description
ACT	Act	Any act of any type
ACCM	Accommodation	Provision of a bed in a ward, or similar activity.
CONS	Consent	A consent to a service (e.g., an operation, or the sharing of information).
CTTEVENT	Clinical Trial Timepoint Event	An identified time where some clinical trial activity is expected to occur.
INC	Incident	An event outside the control of one or more involved (e.g., an accident).
INF	Inform	Communication of information to a person.
PCPR	Care Provision	Taking responsibility for the care of a patient.
REG	Registration	Maintaining information about a subject.
SPCTRT	Specimen Treatment	Preparation of a specimen.

The negationInd class attribute indicates whether the act described is negated. The assumption by the standard when this class attribute is NOT sent is that the act was NOT negated. It should have been assigned a default value of false in the standard because that is the effect of the assumption.

The `text` class attribute represents the text describing the act. In a CDA document, this class attribute is often completed with a reference to the text in the narrative portion of the document, rather than duplicating the actual text. This strategy eliminates an opportunity for introducing errors in the production of the CDA document, since text need not be copied from one place to another.

The `statusCode` class attribute indicates the current state of the act according to the state model for acts described in the HL7 Reference Information model shown in the figure below.

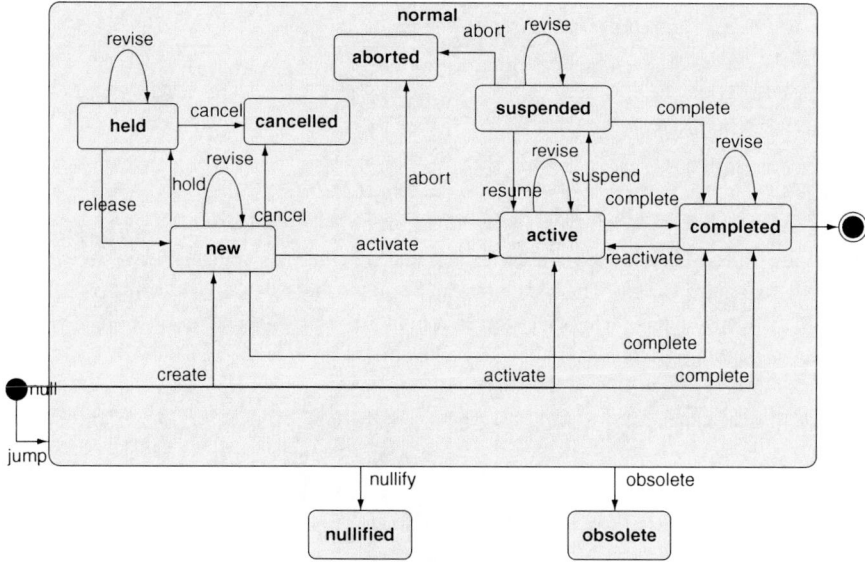

Fig. 16.2 Act states

The most common value used is `completed`, indicating that the act has been completed normally. An act that is still in process will sometimes use `active`. Other act states are used but not commonly in CDA implementations. Most CDA implementations do little examination of the status and simply assume that it is either active (in process) or completed. The use of act status codes such as `aborted`, `nullified`, `obsolete`, `held`, or `suspended` have semantics that are significantly different from `active` or `completed`. Some care should be given to ensure that all parties using CDA to communicate are aware of the act status values that might be present.

The `effectiveTime` class attribute carries the clinically effective time of the act. This may be the time that the act itself performed (e.g., an observation of blood pressure), or it may be a related time. For example, the clinically effective time for a lab result is not when the measurement is performed, but when the specimen that was measured was taken.

The `priorityCode` class attribute indicates the priority in which the act was or is expected to be performed. The HL7 ActPriority vocabulary should be used to specify priority in most cases.

The `languageCode` class attribute specifies the human language in which the act itself is specified. This attribute is rarely used since most CDA implementations are monolingual.

```
<act classCode='ACT' moodCode='EVN' negationInd='false'>
   <id root='…' extension='…'/>
   <code code='…' displayName='…'
      codeSystem='…' codeSystemName='…'/>
   <text><reference value='#IDinCDANarrative'/></text>
   <statusCode code='completed'/>
   <effectiveTime value='…'/>
</act>
```

Fig. 16.3 Act XML example

encounter

The `encounter` class is used to describe acts that are clinical encounters between a healthcare provider and a patient. The encounter can be an inpatient stay, a visit with a consultant, an outpatient encounter, a telephone call, an e-mail message, a video consultation, et cetera. The key is that it be an interaction between a healthcare provider and a patient.

Fig. 16.4 The encounter class

```
Encounter
classCode *: <= ENC
moodCode *: <= x_DocumentEncounterMood
id: SET<II> [0..*]
code: CD CWE [0..1] <=  ActEncounterCode
text: ED [0..1]
statusCode: CS CNE [0..1] <=  ActStatus
effectiveTime: IVL<TS> [0..1]
priorityCode: CE CWE [0..1] <=  ActPriority
```

The class attributes of the `encounter` class are used in the same fashion as for the `act` class. There are really only two distinctions between the `encounter` class and the `act` class in CDA. An encounter cannot be negated (the `negationInd` class attribute is not present). So there is no way to say that a particular type of encounter did not occur using this class.

Also, you cannot define a particular type of encounter in a CDA document, as the `moodCode` class attribute for the `encounter` class does not permit definition (DEF) mood.

```
<encounter classCode='ENC' moodCode='EVN'>
   <id root='…' extension='…'/>
   <code code='…' displayName='…'
      codeSystem='…' codeSystemName='…'/>
   <text><reference value='#IDinCDANarrative'/></text>
   <statusCode code='completed'/>
   <effectiveTime value='…'/>
</encounter>
```

Fig. 16.5 Encounter XML example

procedure

The procedure class is also very much like an act. In the HL7 RIM, a procedure is described as an act whose outcome results in the physical alteration of the subject [§RIM 3.1.15]. This is very different from the idea of activity involved in treatment or diagnosis of disease, but it also provides a very clear distinction of what is and is not a procedure.

Fig. 16.6 Procedure class

```
Procedure
classCode *: <= PROC
moodCode *: <= x_DocumentProcedureMood
id: SET<II> [0..*]
code: CD CWE [0..1]
negationInd: BL [0..1]
text: ED [0..1]
statusCode: CS CNE [0..1] <= ActStatus
effectiveTime: IVL<TS> [0..1]
priorityCode: CE CWE [0..1] <= ActPriority
languageCode: CS CNE [0..1] <= HumanLanguage
methodCode: SET<CE> CWE [0..*]
approachSiteCode: SET<CD> CWE [0..*]
targetSiteCode: SET<CD> CWE [0..*]
```

The procedure class carries the same attributes as the act class and a few more. The methodCode class attribute describes the more detailed method when the code attribute does not fully describe the procedure. Most common uses of procedure do not include this attribute. The approachSiteCode class attribute describes the direction of approach. The targetSiteCode class attribute describes the target of the procedure.

```
<procedure classCode='PROC' moodCode='INT'>
   <id root='…' extension='…'/>
   <code code='…' displayName='…'
       codeSystem='…' codeSystemName='…'/>
   <text><reference value='#IDinCDANarrative'/></text>
   <statusCode code='completed'/>
   <effectiveTime value='…'/>
   <methodCode code='…' displayName='…'
       codeSystem='…' codeSystemName='…'/>
   <approachSiteCode code='…' displayName='…'
       codeSystem='…' codeSystemName='…'/>
   <targetSiteCode code='…' displayName='…'
       codeSystem='…' codeSystemName='…'/>
</procedure>
```

Fig. 16.7 Procedure XML example

observation

The observation class is very similar to the procedure class and can be thought of as a "non-altering" procedure that results in a value. Unlike the procedure class, the observation class does not have an approachSiteCode, but it does have all of the other attributes found in the procedure class.

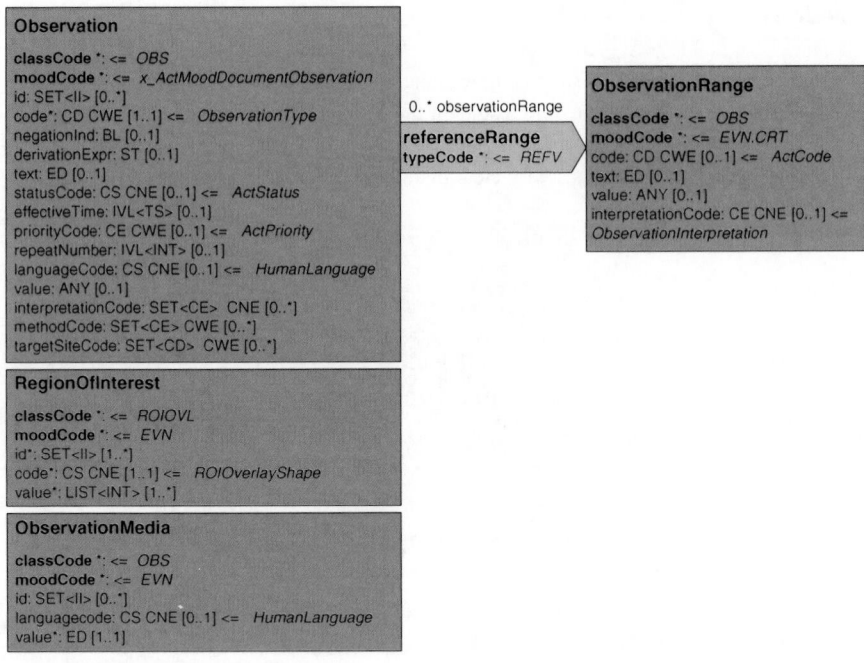

Observation

classCode *: <= *OBS*
moodCode *: <= *x_ActMoodDocumentObservation*
id: SET<II> [0..*]
code*: CD CWE [1..1] <= *ObservationType*
negationInd: BL [0..1]
derivationExpr: ST [0..1]
text: ED [0..1]
statusCode: CS CNE [0..1] <= *ActStatus*
effectiveTime: IVL<TS> [0..1]
priorityCode: CE CWE [0..1] <= *ActPriority*
repeatNumber: IVL<INT> [0..1]
languageCode: CS CNE [0..1] <= *HumanLanguage*
value: ANY [0..1]
interpretationCode: SET<CE> CNE [0..*]
methodCode: SET<CE> CWE [0..*]
targetSiteCode: SET<CD> CWE [0..*]

0..* observationRange

referenceRange
typeCode *: <= *REFV*

ObservationRange

classCode *: <= *OBS*
moodCode *: <= *EVN.CRT*
code: CD CWE [0..1] <= *ActCode*
text: ED [0..1]
value: ANY [0..1]
interpretationCode: CE CNE [0..1] <= *ObservationInterpretation*

RegionOfInterest

classCode *: <= *ROIOVL*
moodCode *: <= *EVN*
id*: SET<II> [1..*]
code*: CS CNE [1..1] <= *ROIOverlayShape*
value*: LIST<INT> [1..*]

ObservationMedia

classCode *: <= *OBS*
moodCode *: <= *EVN*
id: SET<II> [0..*]
languagecode: CS CNE [0..1] <= *HumanLanguage*
value*: ED [1..1]

Fig. 16.8 Observation and related classes

The result of the observation is stored in the `value` class attribute, and can be virtually anything. In fact, because it can be any data type, this class attribute can also be a set, list or bag of information. The resulting value can also have a clinical interpretation (e.g., high, significant, susceptible, et cetera) which can be recorded in the `interpretationCode` class attribute. Although not shown in the diagram, this class attribute is expected to use the HL7 ObservationIntepretation vocabulary. The code values in this vocabulary shown in the table below will be familiar to many HL7 Version 2 interface developers, as these are the same values appearing in OBX-8 Abnormal Flags.

Observations can repeat a number of times. The `repeatNumber` class attribute is used indicate which repetition of the observation is being recorded (e.g., the third blood pressure measurement of the visit).

Table 16.2 Observation interpretation values

Code	Print name	Code	Print name
B	better	I	intermediate
D	decreased	MS	moderately susceptible
U	increased	R	resistant
W	worse	S	susceptible
		VS	very susceptible

Table 16.2 (continued)

Code	Print name	Code	Print name
<	low off scale	>	high off scale
A	Abnormal	N	Normal
AA	Abnormal alert		
HH	High alert	LL	Low alert
H	High	L	Low

```
<observation classCode='OBS' moodCode='EVN'
     negationInd='false'>
  <id root='…' extension='…'/>
  <code code='…' displayName='…'
     codeSystem='…' codeSystemName='…'/>
  <text><reference value='#IDinCDANarrative'/></text>
  <statusCode code='completed'/>
  <effectiveTime value='…'/>
  <value xsi:type='PQ' value='…' unit='…'/>
  <interpretationCode code='H' displayName='High'
     codeSystem='2.16.840.1.113883.5.83'
     codeSystemName='ObservationInterpretation'/>
  <methodCode code='…' displayName='…'
     codeSystem='…' codeSystemName='…'/>
  <targetSiteCode code='…' displayName='…'
     codeSystem='…' codeSystemName='…'/>
  <reference>
     <observationRange>…</observationRange>
  </reference>
</observation>
```

Fig. 16.9 Observation XML example

observationRange

The observationRange class is used to hold values considered to be normal or abnormal for the observation. These are associated with the observation class through the
referenceRange class. In HL7 Version 2, it was common to record the "normal" range
of values for a given observation (in OBX-7 Reference Range). The observation-
Range class can serve that purpose, but it can also identify and classify other range types.
The interpretationCode class attribute indicates what interpretation is associated
with the observationRange class. The text class attribute may give a textual
description of this range.

The value class attribute in the observationRange class should be of the appropriate interval type based on the type of the value in the observation class. If the
value of the observation class is of type PQ, then the value in the observationRange class should be of type IVL_PQ (which is the most common case).

```
<observationRange>
   <code code='…' displayName='…'
      codeSystem='…' codeSystemName='…'/>
   <value xsi:type='PQ' value='…' unit='…'/>
   <interpretationCode code='N' displayName='Normal'
      codeSystem='2.16.840.1.113883.5.83'
      codeSystemName='ObservationInterpretation'/>
</observationRange>
```

Fig. 16.10 observationRange XML example

observationMedia and regionOfInterest

The observationMedia class is a restricted form of the observation class intended to support other forms of media, such as an imaging result. The media can be fully contained in the CDA document and may also be referenced by a renderMultimedia element in the CDA narrative.

The regionOfInterest class is designed to support identification of interesting regions in an image. The interesting regions can be defined as points (POINT), circles (CIRCLE), ellipses (ELLIPSE) or arbitrary polygons (POLY) using this class. The code class attribute indicates which of these region types is being defined. The value attribute is a list of integer pixel locations in the image being overlaid, in X, Y order. Position 0,0 is at the top left of the image, and values increase to the right and towards the bottom of the image.

It has been noted that certain image formats are independent of the size of the viewing window, and so the "pixel" form should be changed to support other data formats. This will likely be addressed in CDA Release 3.

substanceAdministration

The substanceAdministration class is intended to represent the administration of a particular substance, e.g. a medication, immunization or other substance to a patient. The substance may be part of treatment, or it could even represent the exposure of the patient to something they now need to be treated for.

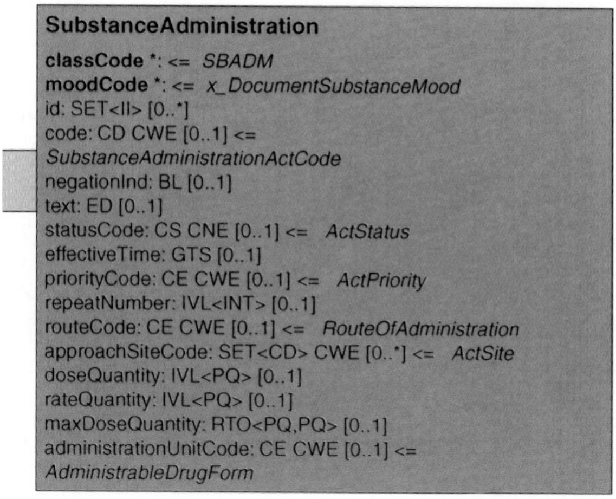

Fig. 16.11 The
SubstanceAdministration
class

```
SubstanceAdministration

classCode *: <= SBADM
moodCode *: <= x_DocumentSubstanceMood
id: SET<II> [0..*]
code: CD CWE [0..1] <=
SubstanceAdministrationActCode
negationInd: BL [0..1]
text: ED [0..1]
statusCode: CS CNE [0..1] <=  ActStatus
effectiveTime: GTS [0..1]
priorityCode: CE CWE [0..1] <=  ActPriority
repeatNumber: IVL<INT> [0..1]
routeCode: CE CWE [0..1] <=  RouteOfAdministration
approachSiteCode: SET<CD> CWE [0..*] <=  ActSite
doseQuantity: IVL<PQ> [0..1]
rateQuantity: IVL<PQ> [0..1]
maxDoseQuantity: RTO<PQ,PQ> [0..1]
administrationUnitCode: CE CWE [0..1] <=
AdministrableDrugForm
```

The substanceAdministation class is very similar to the procedure class, but has additional class attributes and associations to address medication specific information. The consumable association class described in the Sect. 16.3 below (found on page 206) links the substanceAdministration class with the specific medication being given.

code

The code class attribute indicates the kind of substance administration act that was used to administer the substance. The code class attribute is often left out because the route of administration or type of medication usually implies a particular form of administration (e.g., Intravenous vs. Topical or Oral use). The code does not represent the type of substance given, merely the way that it is administered.

routeCode

The routeCode class attribute is used to indicate the route by which the medication (or other substance) is administered. This should be provided and the HL7 RouteOfAdministration vocabulary includes many of the commonly used routes. However, local policy may require the use of certain vocabulary to meet regulatory requirements.

approachSiteCode

The `approachSiteCode` can be used to indicate the site where the medication is administered. An intramuscular injection or a topically applied medication could be administered in a number of different body sites. This class attribute indicates the site where the medication is to be administered. In some cases, it might not be possible to describe the approach site in anything other than text (e.g., apply to area affected by rash). In these cases, you can still use the `approachSiteCode` class attribute, and simply record the description of the site in narrative text using the `originalText` component of the CD data type to record that description. Note that this is actually a set of approach sites, which means that the XML may contain more than one `<approachSiteCode>` elements in the result.

doseQuantity

The `doseQuantity` class attribute allows a range of dosages to be specified, indicating the low and high doses in the range. This class attribute uses the IVL_PQ data type to support this capability. Usually this range is simply collapsed to the single value in the XML.

When the `doseQuantity` being described is for a medication made up of multiple active ingredients (e.g., Acetaminophen with Codeine), the units of the physical quantity should be in dosing units, e.g., tablets or capsules, and the code describing the medication should be specific enough to indicate what a dosing unit is.

rateQuantity

IV medications are often given at a specified rate, rather than a specific dose. This would be provided in the `rateQuantity` class attribute rather than in the `doseQuantity` class attribute. In these cases, one aspect of the PQ in `rateQuantity` must include a time unit in the denominator of the unit expression.

maxDoseQuantity

The dosing regimen may be limited to a maximum dose by storing the maximum dose and for a given period of time in the `maxDoseQuantity` class attribute. This class attribute is particularly useful to provide an overall limit on the dose given, especially when the regimen includes "as needed for ___" instead of a time range between doses.

The `maxDoseQuantity` is specified using the RTO data type, where the numerator is in the dosing quantity and the denominator is units of time. This is different from how `rateQuantity` is specified because `rateQuantity` is assumed to be for continuously divisible fluids (a liquid or a gas), but `maxDoseQuantity` supports indivisible items such as tablets or capsules per day.

administrationUnitCode

The `administrationUnitCode` class attribute is needed for those rare cases where the medication is described as an entire package (e.g., an inhaler or bottle of eyedrops), but the unit of administration is smaller (e.g., an actuation or a drop).

```
<substanceAdministration classCode="SBADM" moodCode="INT">
   <id root="0C2F1384-6C68-4639-A56F-4B654AE809E6"/>
   <text><reference value='#med-1'/></text>
   <statusCode code="completed"/>
   <effectiveTime xsi:type="IVL_TS">
       <low value="20070820"/>
       <high value="20070824"/>
   </effectiveTime>
   <effectiveTime institutionSpecified="true"
       operator="A"
       xsi:type="PIVL_TS">
       <period unit="h" value="8"/>
   </effectiveTime>
   <routeCode code="PO"
       codeSystem="2.16.840.1.113883.5.112"
       codeSystemName="RouteOfAdministration"
       displayName="oral"/>
   <doseQuantity value="1" unit='{tablet}'/>
   <consumable>
   </consumable>
</substanceAdministration>
```

Fig. 16.12 Substance administration XML example

supply

The `supply` class is used to describe things that are given to the patient for their subsequent use, possibly, as in the case of medications, for later administration.

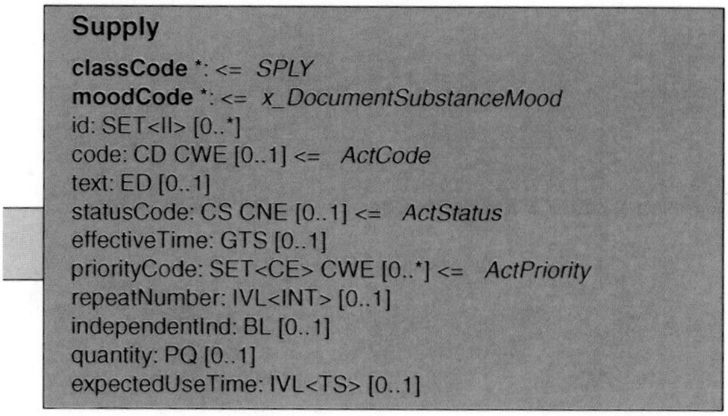

Supply

classCode *: <= SPLY
moodCode *: <= x_DocumentSubstanceMood
id: SET<II> [0..*]
code: CD CWE [0..1] <= ActCode
text: ED [0..1]
statusCode: CS CNE [0..1] <= ActStatus
effectiveTime: GTS [0..1]
priorityCode: SET<CE> CWE [0..*] <= ActPriority
repeatNumber: IVL<INT> [0..1]
independentInd: BL [0..1]
quantity: PQ [0..1]
expectedUseTime: IVL<TS> [0..1]

Fig. 16.13 The Supply class

The supply class is very similar to the procedure class, but has three additional attributes and uses the product association class to link the act with the material being supplied. That association is described in the Sect. 16.3 below (found on page 206.

quantity

The quantity class attribute allows for the number of units of the material being -supplied. This is a physical quantity (data type PQ) that indicates the number of dosing units (where unit is assumed based on the type of material), or as a specific volume, mass or other measurable quantity of the substance.

expectedUseTime

The expectedUseTime class attribute indicates when the material being supplied is expected to be consumed. This is not necessarily the same as the dosing regimen for medications, although it may be related. This is an interval of time (data type IVL_TS) which indicates the time period over which the material could be expected to be used.

```
<supply classCode="SPLY" moodCode="EVN">
   <id root="0C2F1384-6C68-4639-A56F-4B654AE809E7"/>
   <statusCode code="completed"/>
   <effectiveTime value="20070820"/>
   <repeatNumber value="1"/>
   <quantity value="15"/>
</supply>
```

Fig. 16.14 Supply XML example

External Acts

The CDA clinical statement model allows for a clinical statement to refer to external acts, observations, procedures or documents.

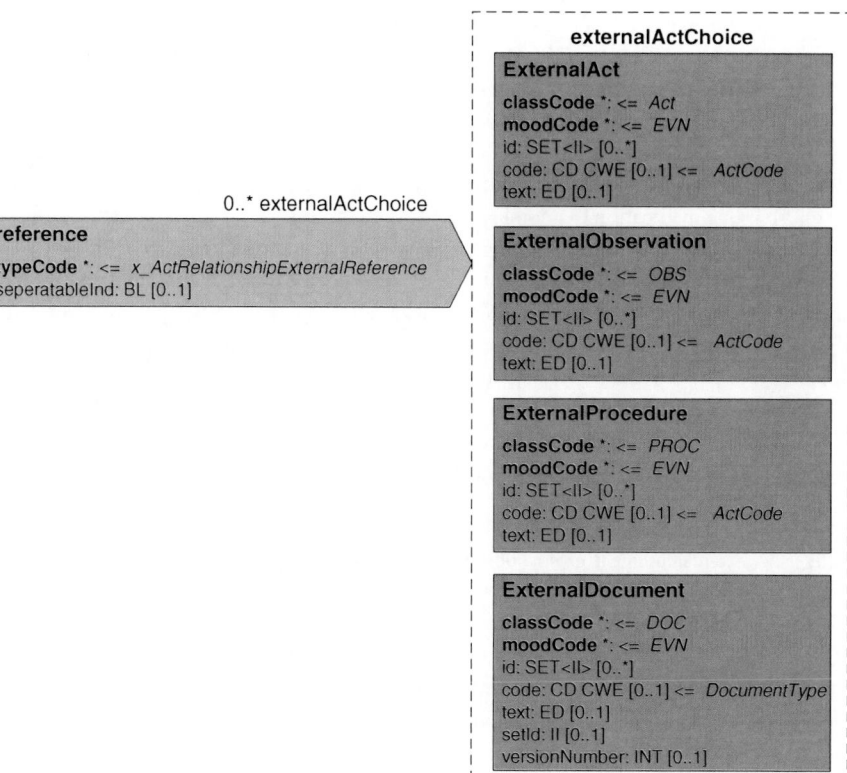

Fig. 16.15 Reference association and related classes

The two acts are linked by the `reference` association class. This association has two attributes.

typeCode

The `typeCode` class attribute describes the relationship between the clinical statement in the CDA document and the external act it references.

The clinical statements in the CDA document can link the current act with the external act to show that the two acts are part of the same "episode" (ELNK). This is only appropriate when the two acts are both observations describing the episode. This draws an equivalence relationship between the two observations indicating that they are related or equivalent with respect to an episode of illness.

In other cases, the act in the CDA document can be designated as a replacement (RPLC) for the external act. In this case, the new act supersedes the information found in the old one. This may represent new information (e.g., a better diagnosis), or a change in treatment (e.g., from one medication to another).

The act in the CDA document could just provide supporting evidence (SPRT) for the external act. The external act could also just be the subject (SUBJ) of commentary found in the CDA document (e.g., a progress note might comment on the patient status after discharge). The weakest relationship is a simple reference (REFR) where there is some link between the two but not really further specified.

In some cases, the act in the CDA document is a summary or excerpt (XCRPT) of the more detailed information found in the external act. This might be the case where only key values from an external lab report are described in the CDA document.

externalAct, externalDocument, externalObservation and externalProcedure

The attributes of all four external acts are nearly identical. The only exception is that the external document can be identified using the id class attribute or the setId and versionNumber class attributes. Most systems use the id class attribute as the principal way to identify clinical documents, so the utility of these latter two attributes seems to be waning.

id

The id class attribute identifies the external act being referenced in some way. While CDA makes this optional, it is hard to indicate an external act without providing some identity for it, so this attribute should usually be sent.

code

The code class attribute further refines the kind of act being referenced. This is not necessary when the external reference is from within a system where the external act is accessible, but CDA documents do not always stay in their "home" system. So it is advisable to fill in the code class attribute if the CDA document making the external reference is ever expected to "leave home".

text

The text class attribute should contain the human readable text of the act being referenced. At the very least this should include text describing the act, observation or procedure. When the reference is to an externalDocument however, treatment of this class attribute is different. The intent of the authors of the CDA standard was to allow the mime type of the external document to be represented, not necessarily duplicating the entire content of the external document. So, the `text` class attribute of the `externalDocument` class should not be used to communicate the entire content of the document. It could however be used to transmit a URL reference to where that content could be accessed. This can be used for example to refer to educational information on the web about patients, diagnoses or test results within a CDA document.

```
<externalDocument>
    <id root='…' extension='…'/>
    <code code='…' displayName='…'
        codeSystem='…' codeSystemName='…'/>
    <text><reference value='https://…'/></text>
</externalDocument>
```

Fig. 16.16 ExternalDocument XML example

Organizer

The `organizer` class is a specialization of the act class that is designed to support grouping of information. The information can be grouped into batteries (e.g., of tests) by assigning the `classCode` attribute a value of BATTERY. In other cases, it can be used to create information structures using the value of CLUSTER. A cluster can contain collections of batteries and individual entries.

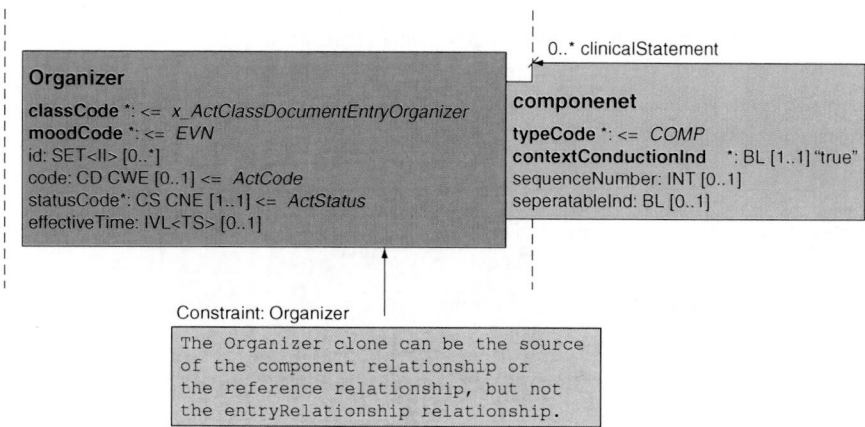

Fig. 16.17 The organizer class

While any act in CDA can be described compositionally, the organizer class is always described compositionally through the `component` associations to other clinical statements. An organizer cannot use any association other than the `component` one with its content, including the `entryRelationship` association.

16.2
EntryRelationship

Any clinical statement class with the exception of the `organizer` class can be associated with another clinical statement via the `entryRelationship` association.

Fig. 16.18 The entryRelationship association class

entryRelationship

typeCode *: <= *x_ActRelationshipEntryRelationship*
inversionInd: BL [0..1]
contextConductionInd   *: BL [1..1] "true"
sequenceNumber: INT [0..1]
negationInd: BL [0..1]
seperatableInd: BL [0..1]

0..* clinicalStatement

This association class allows larger clinical statements to be constructed composition-ally from smaller ones.

typeCode

The `typeCode` class attribute describes the type of association between the two clinical statements. CDA only allows a few of the many possible relationships defined by the RIM, but even this short list creates a broad range of possible clinical statements.

In the following, one class is the *source* of the association, and the other is the *target*. In the XML, the usual direction is from source (outer element) to target (inner element). But the direction of the association can be changed by setting the `inversionInd` class attri-bute to true. If this class attribute is false or not sent, then the relationship follows the usual rules when interpreted from the XML structure.

Table 16.3 Entry relationship types in CDA

Code	Display name	Description
XRCPT	Excerpt	SOURCE summarizes the TARGET.
COMP	Has Component	TARGET is part of SOURCE.
RSON	Has Reason	TARGET is the reason for SOURCE.
SPRT	Has Support	SOURCE observation is supported by TARGET
CAUS	Is Etiology For	SOURCE causes TARGET observation.
GEVL	Evaluates	SOURCE observation evaluates TARGET goal
MFST	Manifestation Of	SOURCE caused by TARGET
REFR	Refers to	SOURCE is related to TARGET

Table 16.3 (continued)

Code	Display name	Description
SAS	Starts after Start of	SOURCE started after TARGET
SUBJ	Has Subject	SOURCE uses TARGET as its subject.

contextConductionInd

This class attribute is usually true (and defaults to that value). It indicates that the context in the XML representation continues to flow through this relationship. This value is often set to false when there are radical changes in context, as might be caused by incorporating clinical statements from different information systems into the CDA document.

sequenceNumber

The sequenceNumber class attribute is often used to represent different components of a larger act in the particular sequence in which they are to be performed. A care plan, for example, might include diagnostic tests and one or more sequential treatments. For example, a care plan for a broken arm, might include imaging, administration of pain killers, setting the bone, application of a cast, additional pain killers, subsequent removal, reimaging and evaluation, and subsequent physical therapy, in that particular order. The sequenceNumber class attribute allows each of the related acts in the care plan to be ordered. Acts that are simultaneous would have the same sequenceNumber.

negationInd

The use of the negationInd class attribute in an entryRelationship class allows one to assert that a particular relationship does not exist between to clinical statements. This can be used to say things like X did not cause Y, or X is not related to Y, or X is not supported by Y. These negatives are useful to rule out particular diagnoses or courses of action in treatment. It is rarely used in many CDA implementations, which also means that there is some danger that the semantics will not be understood by the receiver.

separatableInd

You can separate a car from its wheels without destroying it, but you cannot separate a rose from its petals in the same way. The separatableInd class attribute serves as a flag to indicate those cases where the parts of a clinical statement have NO meaning without the context provided by the larger whole. For example, a severity assessment on a penicillin allergy might indicate that the allergy is severe. But the clinical statement alone providing the assessment would only say "the assessment of an unknown subject act" is severe, which is meaningless without the subject act. If the target act cannot stand by itself without knowledge of the source act, then this class attribute should be set to false.

```
<entryRelationship typeCode='SUBJ' inversionInd='true'
   negationInd='false'
>
   <sequenceNumber value='…'/>
   <separatableInd value='false'/>
   <!-- A Clinical statement -->
   <act>…</act>
</entryRelationship>
```

Fig. 16.19 EntryRelationship XML example

16.3
Participants

Consumable and Product

The consumable association class connects a manufacturedProduct to a substanceAdministration class. The product association class connects the manufacturedProduct class to a supply class.

The consumable and product association classes most often associate the medications or vaccinations administered or given with the appropriate substanceAdministration or supply activity. The supply class can also be used to associate the supply class some other sort of manufactured material such as a medical device (You rarely if ever "administer" a medical device to a patient).

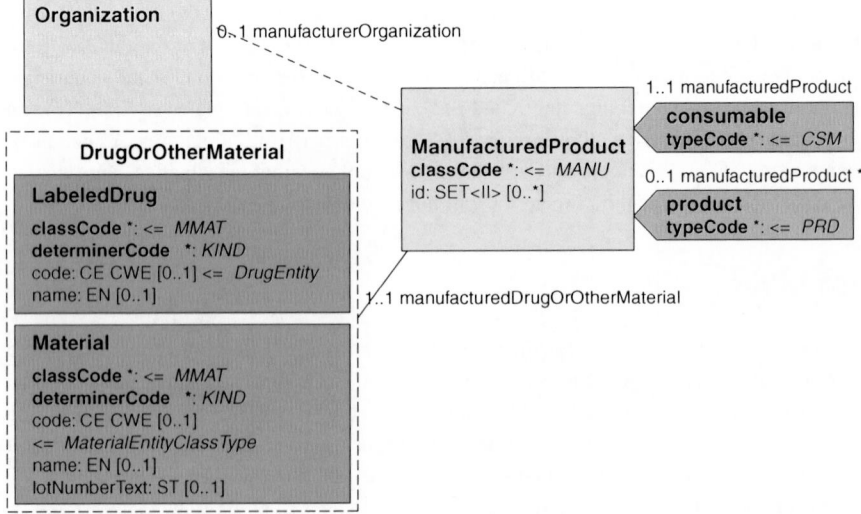

Fig. 16.20 The consumable and product association classes

These associations use the `ManufacturedProduct` class to point to a class representing a manufactured material, or more specifically a labeled drug. The `id` class attribute can be used to provide a unique identifier for the material provided. In the case of a medical device, this could be the device serial number.

The only semantic differences between the `Material` and the `LabeledDrug` class is that the `Material` class supports a broader set of `code` class attributes, and can identify a specific lot of materials in the `lotNumberText` class attribute. The `LabeledDrug` class is intended for medications, but `lotNumberText` is also relevant to medications, and so `Material` is often used instead of `LabeledDrug` in many cases. Given the choices and capabilities of the two classes, I would recommend use of `Material` class in all cases.

The `manufacturerOrganization` class attribute points to the organization that manufactured the medication. It follows the same pattern as other organization classes in the CDA standard.

```
<consumable> <-- OR --> <product>
    <manufacturedProduct>
        <manufacturedMaterial>
          <code code="260448"
              codeSystem="2.16.840.1.113883.6.88"
              codeSystemName="RxNorm"
              displayName="Acetaminophen 300 MG / Codeine
60 MG Oral Tablet [Tylenol with Codeine #4]"/>
              <name>Tylenol #4</name>
        </manufacturedMaterial>
        <manufacturerOrganization>
            ...
        </manufacturerOrganization>
    </manufacturedProduct>
</consumable> <-- OR --> </product>
```

Fig. 16.21 Consumable and product XML examples

Participant

The generic `participant` class in the CDA Clinical Statement model offers even more flexibility than the similarly named class in the CDA Header.

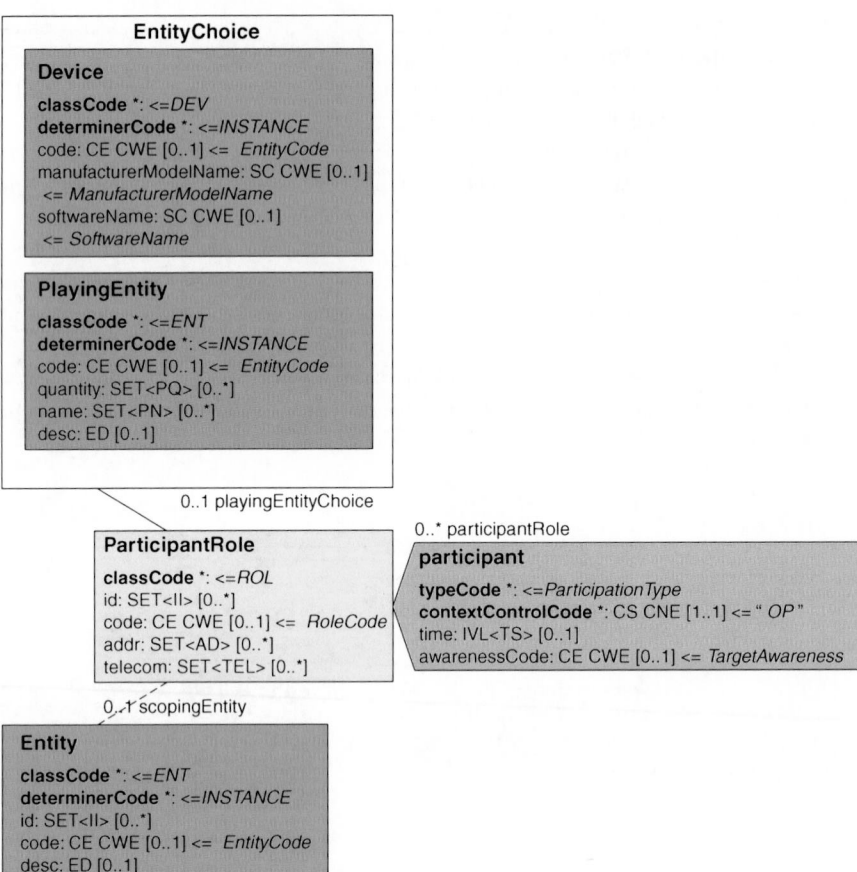

Fig. 16.22 The participant association and related classes

Unlike the participant class in the CDA header, the participant class in the CDA Clinical Statement model records the awareness of the participation in the awarenessCode class attribute. This can be used to indicate for example, that a related family member is or is not aware of a particular health issue that may be indicated by the clinical statement with which they are associated through the participant class.

The participant class in the CDA clinical statement model is also not limited to people as it might be in the CDA header. Thus, the participantRole class does not necessarily indicate the role of a person. This leads to the different name for the role class associated with the clinical statement. Even so, the id, code, addr and telecom class attributes of the participantRole class have the same meaning as the similarly named attributes of the associatedEntity class described previously.

The key difference is that the participantRole allows the playing entity to be any kind of entity (via the PlayingEntity class), or more specifically, a Device using the Device class. When the player of the role uses the PlayingEntity class, its name and description can be provide in the name and desc class attributes. When the player of the role uses the Device class, the model and software names can be provided in the manufacturerModelName and softwareName class attributes.

```
<participant typeCode="IND">
   <time value='0'/>
   <awarenessCode/>
   <participantRole classCode="AGNT">
       <id root='…' extension='…'/>
       <code code='…' displayName='…'
           codeSystem='…' codeSystemName='…'/>
       <addr>…</addr>
       <telecom value='…'/>
       <playingDevice>
           <code …/>
           <manufacturerModelName>…</manufacturerModelName>
           <softwareName>…</softwareName>
       </playingDevice>
       <playingEntity>
           <code …/>
           <quantity value='…' unit='…'/>
           <name>…</name>
           <desc>…</name>
       </playingEntity>
       <scopingEntity>
           <id root='…' extension='…'/>
           <code …/>
           <desc>…</name>
       </scopingEntity>
   </participantRole>
</participant>
```

Fig. 16.23 Clinical statement participant XML example

performer

The performer association class connects the performer of an act to the role of the person performing the act. This class is almost exactly like the performer association in the Service event found in the CDA Header (see page 140). The only differences between this class in the Clinical Statement model and the similarly named participant association class in the CDA header is that it lets the mode of participation be recorded in the modeCode class attribute, and does not support the functionCode class attribute.

specimen

The specimen class associates a clinical statement with the specimenPlayingEntity class through specimenRole class. It is typically associated with a procedure or observation class. In the former case, the specimen is often produced as a product of the procedure (e.g., a biopsy). In the latter case, the specimen is the subject of the observation. The specimen participation is defined by the HL7 Vocabulary to be a subtype of the subject participation.

Fig. 16.24 Specimen classes

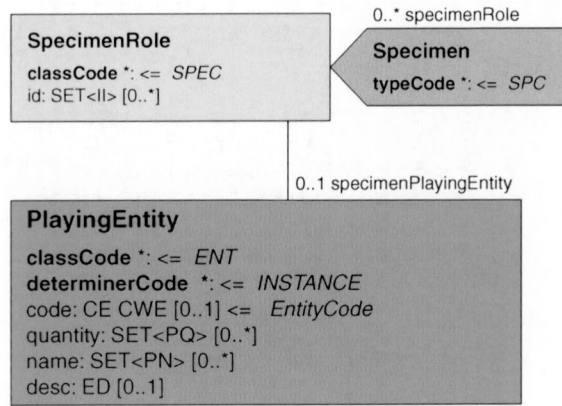

The `specimenRole` class is almost fully defined by CDA. The only implementation supplied value is the identifier of the specimen, which appears in the `id` class attribute on the `specimenRole` class.

The `specimenPlayingEntity` is a very generic entity which can describe any kind of specimen. The `code` class attribute describes the type of specimen. The physical quantity of the specimen can be recorded in the quantity class attribute (e.g., by weight, size or volume).

```
<specimen>
   <specimenRole>
       <id root='…' extension='…'/>
       <specimenPlayingEntity>
           <code code='…' displayName='…'
               codeSystem='…' codeSystemName='…'/>
           <quantity value='…' unit='…'/>
           <name>…</name>
           <desc>…</name>
       </specimenPlayingEntity>
   </specimenRole>
</specimen>
```

Fig. 16.25 Specimen XML example

Summary

- The Clinical Statement model is used to write machine readable clinical statements.
- Clinical statements elements can be connected to each other by `entryRelationship` association classes.
- The `act` class is the foundation for all the other classes.

- The `text` class attribute should reference text in the narrative rather than copy it to avoid possible logic errors in duplication.
- The `effectiveTime` class attribute indicates the clinical relevant time, which may be different from when the activity related to the act occurred.
- HL7 defines an encounter as an interaction between a healthcare provider and a patient. It does now specify how or where it can occur.
- According to the HL7, a procedure results in the physical alteration of the subject.
- Observations are like procedures (from an engineering perspective) with the addition of a result.
- The value class attribute of an observation class can be in any HL7 data type.
- Observations can be associated with variety of normal or abnormal ranges using the `observationRange` class.
- The `observationMedia` and `regionOfInterest` classes allow images and other multi-media objects to be part of the clinical document, and highlights on different parts of these objects to be rendered.
- The `substanceAdministration` class represents the administration of medications or immunizations to a patient.
- The `supply` class describes what has been given to a patient for later use.
- There are four nearly identical classes representing external acts.
- The `externalDocument` class represents a related document that referenced by, but not part of the CDA instance.
- The `organizer` class is used to create collections of related information components, much like a class or data structure in common object oriented programming languages.
- The `consumable` and `product` associations are used to associate `substanceAdministration` and `supply` classes with the relevant medications or other materials.
- The generic `participant` association class in the clinical statement model can be used to associate a clinical statement with people, places or things.
- The `performer` association class connects an act with the person performing it.
- The `specimen` association class connects an act with the specimen that is related to that act.

Questions

1. What clinical statement class is the basis for all others?
2. How can you determine if an act should be represented as a procedure?
3. How is an observation like a procedure? How is it different?
4. What class can be use to group a collection of related observations together?
5. How would you indicate that a medication is being used to treat a particular condition?
6. How would you associate a medication with the act of treating the patient with it? In what way would this differ from giving the medication to the patient for them to use subsequently?

7. What class attribute would you need to use to indicate that a patient had not been diagnosed with a particular illness?
8. What class attribute would you need to use to indicate that the cause of a reaction was not the administration of a particular medication?

Research Questions

1. What other HL7 Standards use the clinical statement model?
2. How does there clinical statement model differ from the one present in CDA?

A very common way to generate CDA documents is by converting an HL7 Version 2 message into the CDA format. The MDM, ORU and ADT messages are the most common ones that are converted to CDA.

Converting these messages is fairly straightforward. There is a three step process:

1. Map message segments and fields into the CDA Structures
2. Map HL7 V2 user and standard code tables into HL7 Version 3 vocabularies.
3. Assign Object Identifiers (OIDS) to the various identifiers in the CDA document.

These mappings can be performed by most interface engines, but the mapping process in those engines is often very tedious. A better way is to convert the HL7 Version 2 message into its XML equivalent, and then apply an XSL transformation to convert the generated XML into the CDA format. Several interface engines can automatically convert from the HL7 EDIFACT message format (the message using | and ^ delimiters) into an XML format. One or two might even support the HL7 Standard XML formats for Version 2 messages, but if they don't, simply use the XML provided by your interface engine.

Note that few people are aware that there are XML formats for HL7 Version 2 messages. XML formats have been defined for all editions of the HL7 Version 2 standard. The XML encoding of Version 2 messages was standardized by HL7 in 2003 in the HL7 Version 2: XML Encoding Syntax, Release 1 Standard.

Mappings in this chapter are based on the definitions in the HL7 Version 2.3.1 standard, that being both the most common HL7 version in use, and the most practical source material to work with. HL7 Version 2.3.1 was the last edition of HL7 Version 2 to be delivered in a single document. Since then the material has been delivered as a collection of chapters. The only exception to in this chapter is for the mapping for the SPM segment, which appeared for the first time in HL7 Version 2.5 standard.

There is a great deal of duplication between the ORC and OBR segments, and the ORB and SPM segments. Some of the mappings below direct you to the same locations in the CDA XML because of this duplication.

The mappings in this book should be considered instructive rather than authoritative. The mappings for ORU messages are loosely based on the IHE XD-Lab profile and the HL7 Laboratory Result message. As a general rule, you should use published guides from consensus based standards and profiling bodies as the authoritative resources.

K.W. Boone, *The CDA™ Book*,
DOI: 10.1007/978-0-85729-336-7_17, © Springer-Verlag London Limited 2011

This chapter contains a number of CDA examples which shows how information in the HL7 Version 2 message segment would be mapped to the CDA XML, as shown in the figure below.

```
<assignedEntity>
    <id root='…' extension='OBX-15.1'/>
    <assignedPerson>
```

Fig. 17.1 Mapping Version 2 to CDA

The example shows a skeleton of the CDA XML with the fields or components of the segment in italics where the information they contain will be mapped to the document. The information to be mapped is usually a field from a segment, in which case it appears in the form *XXX-FF*, where XXX represents the segment name, and FF represents the index of the field in the segment. In a few cases, as in the example above, the form will be *XXX-FF.C* where the last part C represents the component in the field.

In some cases, the information from these fields or components can be copied directly into the CDA XML. In others, it requires further translation. For example, values from HL7 Version 2 code tables may need to be converted into a different vocabulary, or the identifier namespace may need to be set.

These examples are skeletal. They do not include every XML element required or allowed by CDA, nor do they include all the necessary attributes.

MDM Message

In MDM messages, a single OBX segment often carries the entire contents of the document. This segment can be plain text, rich text (e.g., RTF), or content in some other format (e.g., PDF or a proprietary word processing format). In other cases, multiple OBX segments are present, where each OBX segment represents a separate line or section of text in the document.

In cases where a single OBX is used, new lines are most often represented by using repeated OBX-5 components (using the repeat character, usually a tilde ~). They can also be represented using a hexadecimal escape sequence (in the form \X0D\ or \X0A\ or both). More often than not, line breaks are inserted to support a fixed line width (e.g., 65 or 78 characters), with word wrapping enabled. Documents displayed using these line breaks can appear choppy. Some systems insert a double line break to indicate a true line break, and a single line break to end each line of text at a reasonable line width. You may have to experiment, or better yet explore the documentation, design or implementation of the outbound document interface to determine how to best craft the text.

When formats other than plain text, such as RTF or PDF are used, the OBX-2 field will often use the HL7 Version 2 ED data type. Like the HL7 Version 3 data type of the same name, this Version 2 data type allows the contents to be base-64 encoded, and can record a specific MIME type for the data. In these cases, the content of the document is best represented in CDA using a `<NonXMLBody>` element where the `<text>` content is stored in exactly the same form as it is in the HL7 Version 2 message.

More structured report forms may use several OBX segments, where each OBX segment represents a separate part of the document. This is typical in imaging reports, where one OBX might record the impressions, and another the recommendations. In these cases, each OBX might be recorded as a separate `<section>` in a `<structuredBody>` element in the CDA document. Chapter 8 of the HL7 Version 2 standard provides some guidelines on how the different parts of narrative reports are coded in the section titled *Narrative reports as batteries with many OBX* in the HL7 Version 2 standards.

ADT Messages

In ADT messages, OBX segments are typically used to represent specific kinds of information in a name/value pair representation. The OBX-3 field contains a code that explains the value that appears in OBX-5 and OBX-6. These segments are typically used to record common observations like vital signs, height and weight. They may also be used to represent strings or coded values for things like chief complaint, reason for visit, et cetera.

Information items might be grouped or not in the resulting output depending on the organization's business needs. Vital signs, height and weight values might be recorded in a table in a vital signs section in the CDA document, and other name/value pairs such as chief complaint and reason for visit could be recorded in separate sections using narrative text.

ORU Messages

OBX segments appearing in an ORU message use both the single-OBX form found in MDM messages, and can also use the name/value pair structure found in ADT messages.

Laboratory reports (except pathology) and diagnostic studies that typically result in tabular reports of numerical measurements (EKG, fetal ultrasound) often take the name/value form (and may include a narrative interpretation section).

Imaging studies and pathology tests more often have a narrative form.

ORU messages allow multiple OBX segments to be associated with an OBR segment. The OBR segment indicates the requested observation(s), and the OBX segments beneath an OBR report the results of the requested observation. In these cases, each OBR can represent a single section of the CDA document.

Common Message Segments

A number of message elements are common to two or more of these messages. This includes the MSH, EVN, PID, PD1, PV1, PV2, and OBX segments. Having created a conversion from one of these segments to CDA, you can often use it in other conversions. The OBX segment requires care because it is used in different ways in messages.

The table below shows the mapping of HL7 Version 2 segments to XML elements in the CDA document.

Table 17.1 HL7 Version 2 segment to CDA mapping

V2	CDA XML element	V2	CDA XML element
OBX	`<observation>` `<nonXMLBody>`	MSH/EVN	`<ClinicalDocument>`
TXA	`<ClinicalDocument>`	ORC	`<infulfillmentOf>`
PID	`<recordTarget>`	OBR	`<section>` `<observation>`
PV1	`<encompassingEncounter>`	NTE	`<text>`
NK1	`<participant>`	SPM	`<specimen>` `<procedure>`

17.1
HL7 Version 2 Data Type Mappings

Many HL7 Version 2 data types have very simple mappings to HL7 Version 3 data types. The table shows the Version 3 equivalents.

Table 17.2 Version 2 to Version 3 data type mappings

Version 2	Version 3	Version 2	Version 3
AD	ADDR	ID	CS, CD
CE, CNE, CWE	CD	HD	OID, UUID
CN	II + PN	NM	REAL, PQ
CK, CX, EI	II	PN, XPN	PN
DT, TS	TS	RP	TEL
ED	ED	TN, XTN	TEL

The following sections address the most commonly used mappings.

AD – Address

The Version 2 address data type can be mapped into the HL7 Version 3 ADDR datatype. The components of the AD data type are mapped as shown in the figure below. The seventh component of the AD data type should be mapped into the appropriate value for the use XML attribute on the `<addr>` element.

```
<addr use='AD.7'>
   <!-- Line breaks included for clarity,
        See the ADDR data type for proper formatting -->
   <streetAddressLine>AD.1</streetAddressLine>
   <streetAddressLine>AD.2</streetAddressLine>
   <city>AD.3</city>
   <state>AD.4</state>
   <postalCode>AD.5</postalCode>
   <country>AD.6</country>
   <county>AD.8</county>
</addr>
```

Fig. 17.2 AD to HL7 addr mapping

CE – Coded Element, CNE – Coded No Exceptions, CWE – Coded With Exceptions

The CE data type supports the identification of two codes, a primary code which should be a universal one (e.g., from a standard), and an alternate which may be the local code. This maps to the HL7 Version 3 CD data type or its subtypes. The third and sixth components will often have to be mapped to the appropriate `codeSystem` XML attribute via a table lookup. The CNE data type extends from CE and adds code system version and original text components. The CWE data type has the same structure as the CNE data type in Version 2. The mapping of these data types to a code element is shown below.

```
<code code='CE.1' displayName='CE.2'
   codeSystemName='CE.3' codeSystem='CE.3'
   codeSystemVersion='CNE.7'>
   <originalText>CNE.9</originalText>
   <translation code='CE.4' displayName='CE.5'
      codeSystemName='CE.6' codeSystem='CE.6'
      codeSystemVersion='CNE.8'/>
</code>
```

Fig. 17.3 CE to CDA code mapping

CN – Composite ID Number and Name

Many message segments make use of the HL7 CN, XCN or PPN Data Type. The field that this is contained in will identify the appropriate participations and roles of the person in the CDA document. These data types contain the identifier of the person in the first component of the field. This value goes into the `<id>` element of the role, usually an `<assigne-dEntity>` element. Components 2 through 7 would appear in `<family>`, `<given>`, `<given>` (middle), `<suffix>`, `<prefix>` and `<suffix qualifier='AC'>` elements of the `<name>` element of the `<assignedPerson>`. The example shown below indicates how the XCN data type appearing in field OBX-15 would be placed into an `<assignedEntity>` in a CDA document.

```
<assignedEntity>
   <id root='…' extension='OBX-15.1'/>
   <assignedPerson>
      <!-- line breaks included for clarity.
           See PN data type for appropriate formatting.
      -->
      <name>
         <prefix>OBX-15.6</prefix>
         <given>OBX-15.3</given>
         <given>OBX-15.4</given>
         <family>OBX-15.2</family>
         <suffix>OBX-15.5</suffix>
         <suffix qualifier='AC'>OBX-15.7</suffix>
      </name>
   </assignedPerson>
</assignedEntity>
```

This pattern is followed in almost all cases where XCN or PPN is used. Note that the example above uses a western ordering for name components. This will not be appropriate in all regions of the world.

CK, CX – Composite ID with Check Digit

The CK and CX data types are identifiers, which may or may not contain a check digit. This data type is often used to transmit the identifier of a person or organization in HL7 Version 2 messages. The mapping from these data types to an HL7 Version 3 II data type often requires a table lookup on the fourth component of the CK or CX data type, or use of a fixed value depending upon the interface implementation. See also HD below.

```
<id root='CK.4'
   assigningAuthorityName='CK.4.1'
   extension='CK.1'/>
```

Fig. 17.4 CK and CX data types mapped to a CDA id element

DT – Date and TS – TimeStamp

Dates and Timestamps map to the HL7 Version 3 TS Data type. The HL7 Version 2 DT date data type is simply a truncated form of the Version 2 TS data type. The value in the Date or Timestamp be copied without modification into the value XML attribute of the <time> or <effectiveTime> elements (or its <low> or <high> components).

ED – Encapsulated Data

The ED data type in HL7 Version 2 serves the same purpose as the ED data type in Version 3. The second component of the ED data type identifies the MIME type of the content. The third component identifies the MIME subtype. The fourth component is either A, Hex, or Base64 to identify the encoding used for the data. The fifth component is the encapsulated data itself. The figure below shows how a Version 2 ED data type can be mapped into a Version 3 ED data type.

```
<value xsi:type='ED' mediaType='ED.2/ED.3'
   representation='ED.4'>ED.5</value>
```

Fig. 17.5 ED mapping from Version 2 to CDA

EI – Entity Identifier

The entity identifier is another form of identifier similar to the CK and CX data types, save that it does not contain a check digit.

```
<id root='EI.3'
   assigningAuthorityName='EI.3.1'
   extension='EI.1'/>
```

Fig. 17.6 EI data type mapped to a CDA id element

ID – Coded Value for HL7 Tables and IS – Coded Value for User Defined Tables

The HL7 Version 2 ID and IS data types are most like the Version 3 CS data type used to represent content with fixed coding systems. These often need to be mapped to new vocabularies in CDA, and so are mapped to a CD data type (or subtype) by lookup.

HD – Hierarchical Descriptor

The HD data type represents an assigning authority for identifiers, and is often used as a component of other data types containing identifiers. The first component of the HD is a string used as a namespace identifier. This can be mapped directly into the assigning authority name. Usually the XML `root` attribute of an II data type needs to be determined by lookup on this component. If the second and third components are present, they provide an alternate means of ensuring unique assigning authority descriptors. The second component is some form of unique ID, and the third component is the type of unique identifier used for the assigning authority. If the third component contains the code GUID, UUID or ISO, then the second component can be used directly in the root XML attribute of the II data type. Otherwise the root XML attribute needs to be looked up based on either the contents of HD.1 or a combination of HD.2 and HD.3.

```
<id root='CK.4.2'
   assigningAuthorityName='CK.4.1'
   extension='…'/>
```

Fig. 17.7 Use of HD with the II data type

NM – Numeric

The NM data type should most often be mapped to a PQ in CDA, because it is often accompanied by a unit designation in the same field. By itself it is simple a real number and can be mapped to the HL7 Version 3 INT or REAL data types.

PN – Person Name

The HL7 Version 2 PN data type is mapped to the data type of the same name in Version 3. The mapping is very similar to that shown for CN, save that the ID number component is missing, so all fields are shifted down by one.

```
<name>
   <prefix>CN.5</prefix>
   <given>CN.3</given>
   <given>CN.4</given>
   <family>CN.2</family>
   <suffix>CN.5</suffix>
   <suffix qualifier='AC'>CN.7</suffix>
</name>
```

RP – Reference Pointer

The RP data type is used to access data by reference instead of by value. The Version 3 ED data type supports this type of reference. The first component identifies the data to be referenced, and the second component the system from which it can be obtained. These two components will need to be mapped into some form of URL.

```
<value xsi:type='ED' mediaType='RP.2/RP.3'><reference
value='RP.1 and RP.2'/></value>
```

TN – Telephone Number and XTN – Extended Telecommunication Number

The Version 2 TN data type is mapped to the TEL data type in HL7 Version 3. The XTN data type can actually contain both a telephone number and an e-mail address and so may need to be mapped to two TEL data elements. While XTN breaks the phone number up into several parts, most systems using it still only send the number in the first component. The TN and XTN data types record a two digit country code (*NN* below), ten dialing digits (9999999999 below) and up to a five digit extension (XXXXX below) in the first component. If the country code is not present, it must be supplied by the mapping. The second component of the XTN data type should be mapped to the appropriate value for the use XML attribute.

```
<telecom value='tel:+NN9999999999;ext=XXXXX' use='XTN.2'>
```

Fig. 17.8 TN to CDA telecom mapping

XTN can also contain an e-mail address in the fourth component.

```
<telecom value='mailto:XTN.4' use='XTN.2'>
```

Fig. 17.9 XTN to CDA telecom mapping

17.2
Converting Codes and Assigning Authorities

In the mappings for data types given above, you will need to somehow determined what OIDs to use for the various identifiers that have been mapped. In most cases the interface containing the message to be mapped will use identifiers from fixed "assigning authorities", and so the mappings of the root XML attribute in the various <id> elements in the converted CDA document can be pre-computed. However, there are times when you might be receiving for example, laboratory results from multiple laboratories on a single inbound interface. In these cases you will need to determine how to map the root XML attribute for each of the identifiers that are generated.

One way to accomplish this is to use the HD (Hierarchical Descriptor) component of the field containing the identifier. The first component of the HD contains a string representing an assigning authority. This should be mapped into the appropriate OID representing that identifier namespace. One way to accomplish this is by table lookup.

A similar problem occurs when mapping from local code systems to standard codes. Often you can create a one to one mapping from the codes appearing in the interface to a standards based code (e.g., LOINC or SNOMED CT). This is especially true in mapping from many HL7 Version 2 tables to HL7 Version 3 value sets (e.g., for race, gender, ethnicity, marital status, religion, et cetera).

If you are using XSLT to transform an XML representation of the HL7 Version 2 message, table lookups can be accomplished by a very simple XSLT technique. You can create a variable containing the contents of an external document in your stylesheet as follows:

```
<xsl:variable name='lookup'
    select='document("lookup-table.xml")'/>
```

Later, if you want to find a particular element from that document, you can access it using an XPath expression.

```
<xsl:variable name='code' select='./OBX-3'/>
<xsl:variable name='mappedCode'
    select='$lookup//mapping[@original=$code]/@new'/>
```

In the example above, the first statement stores value of the <OBX-3> element in the code variable. The second statement finds the first <mapping> element in the document loaded into the lookup variable where the original XML attribute matches the code found in the <OBX-3> above. The result is returned in the mappedCode variable. This is a very simple technique that can used to map either codes or namespace descriptors to the appropriate values in an XSLT stylesheet. This technique can be extended to match on more than one attribute in the <mapping> element to map from different coding systems, or different parts of a hierarchical descriptor.

17.3
Observation (OBX)

The OBX segment appears in ADT, ORU and MDM messages. The conversion of an OBX segment is highly dependent on the data type that appears in it, the type of message it appears in, and organizational policies and procedures for how the segment is created for each message type. There are no hard and fast rules, only heuristics, which follow.

There are two general forms. The narrative OBX form includes a code in OBX-3 which describes the text found in OBX-5. These observations map most closely to a CDA <section> element. The code in OBX-3 maps to a <code> element in the <section>, and the text in OBX-5 would appear in the <text> element of the CDA <section>.

The name/value form also includes a code in OBX-3, but uses a numeric, timestamp or coded data type appearing in OBX-5. These most closely map to the CDA <observation> element. Again, the code in OBX-3 would appear in a <code> element. The value in OBX-5 maps to the <value> element of the <observation>, and the appropriate data type should be specified for the <value> element.

```
<observation>
    <code code='OBX-3' …/>
    <value xsi:type='OBX-2' value='OBX-5' unit='OBX-6'/>
    <effectiveTime value='OBX-14'/>
    <interpretationCode code='OBX-8'
        codeSystem='2.16.840.1.113883.5.83'
        codeSystemName='ObservationInterpretation'/>
    <methodCode code='OBX-17'/>
    <author>
        <assignedAuthor>
            <id root='…' extension='OBX-16.1'/>
            <authorPerson>
                <name>OBX-16.2 - OBX-16.8</name>
            </authorPerson>
        </assignedAuthor>
    </author>
    <performer>
        <assignedEntity>
            <id root='…' extension='OBX-15.1'/>
            <assignedPerson>
                <name>OBX-15.2 - OBX-15.8</name>
            </assignedPerson>
        </assignedEntity>
    </performer>
    <referenceRange>
        <observationRange>
            <code code='OBX-10' …/>
            <value xsi:type='IVL_OBX-2' unit='OBX-6'>
                <low value='OBX-7'/>
                <high value='OBX-7'/>
            </value>
            <observationInterpretation
                code='N' displayName='normal'
                codeSystem='2.16.840.1.113883.5.83'
                codeSystemName='ObservationInterpretation'
            />
        </observationRange>
    </referenceRange>
</observation>
```

Fig. 17.10 OBX to CDA observation mapping

```
<component>
   <section>
      <code code='OBX-3'/>
      <text>OBX-5</text>
      <author>See author in previous figure</author>
      <entry>
         <observation>See previous figure</observation>
      </entry>
   </section>
</component>
```

Fig. 17.11 OBX to CDA section Mapping

Value Type (OBX-2)

An OBX Segment can contain just about any kind of value on the OBX-5 field. The OBX-2 field indicates the type of data contained in OBX-5. Many interface engines do not correctly handle the value-type variations and treat all OBX-5 fields as containing a string value. This means that your application will often have to parse the components from the OBX-5 field if something other than HL7 Version 2 ST data type is used (e.g., a code item using the CE data type).

The table below shows the mapping of common HL7 Version 2 data types to the Version 3 data types used by the CDA standard. When storing OBX segments in an <observation> element, this mapping is needed to determine how to specify the data type for the value element. If, for example

Table 17.3 Common HL7 Version 2 data types mapped to Version 3 data types

Type	Name	CDA type	Example
ST	String	ST	`<value xsi:type='ST'>` ... `</value>`
ED	Encapsulated Data	ED	`<value xsi:type='ED'>` ... `</value>`
NM	Numeric	PQ	`<value xsi:type='PQ' value='...' unit='...'>`
CE	Coded Value	CD	`<value xsi:type='CD' code='...' codeSystem='...' />`
TS	Timestamp	TS	`<value xsi:type='TS' value='...' >`

Observation Identifier (OBX-3)

This field can contain a code and an alternate. Each code can have an identifier (the code), a display name or text representation, and a code system name. Many systems send only one code (and a local code at that), even though the HL7 recommends the use of universal (or standard) codes such as LOINC and SNOMED CT. In narrative forms, these codes are indicate the `<code>` appearing in the `<section>` (e.g., chief complaint, reason for visit). In name/value forms they identify the `<code>` for the `<observation>` made.

When both a code and an alternate are present in OBX-3, one can be placed in the `<code>` element and the other in a `<translation>` element beneath the `<code>`. Determining which code goes where in the CDA instance needs to be determined based on business rules.

Observation Subidentifier (OBX-4)

The observation subidentifier is used to distinguish between different OBX segments. If two OBX segments have the same subidentifier, they are part of the same group. In these cases, the observations can be grouped together in the CDA instance using the `<organizer>` element, with the actual values being placed in `<observation>` elements that appear inside different `<component>` elements of the `<organizer>`.

Observation Value (OBX-5)

This field contains the results of the observation. In narrative forms, this would appear in the `<text>` element of the `<section>`. In name/value forms it would appear in the `<value>` element of the `<observation>`.

Observation Units (OBX-6)

This field contains the units that the observation was measured in and is most often used when the data type in OBX-2 is NM (Numeric). Mapping the HL7 Version 2 unit field into CDA requires converting from the ISO+ units supported by the HL7 Version 2 standard to UCUM.

The following mapping was produced for the HL7 Claims Attachments implementation guides but was never used. I later published it on the web at http://bit.ly/ISO2UCUM. The current mapping tables at the time of this publication appear below.

Table 17.4 ISO+ to UCUM mapping

ISO+	UCUM	ISO+	UCUM
(arb_u)	[arb'U]	iu/L	[iU]/L
(bdsk_u)	[bdsk'U]	iu/min	[iU]/min
(bsa)	{bsa}	iu/mL	[iU]/mL
(cal)	cal	k/watt	K/W
(cfu)	{cfu}	kg(body_wt)	kg{body_wt}
(drop)	[drp]	kg/ms	kg/m^2
(ka_u)	[ka'U]	kh/h	kg/h
(kcal)	kcal	L/(8.hr)	L/(8.h)
(kcal)/(8.hr)	kcal/(8.h)	L/hr	L/h
(kcal)/d	kcal/d	lb	[lb_av]
(kcal)/hr	kcal/h	mas	Ms
(knk_u)	[knk'U]	m/s	ms/s
(mclg_u)	[mclg'U]	meq/(8.hr)	meq/(8.h)
(od)	{od}	meq/(8.hr.kg)	meq/(8.h.kg)
(ph)	pH	meq/(kg.hr)	meq/(kg.h)
(ppb)	[ppb]	meq/hr	meq/h
(ppm)	[ppm]	mg/(8.hr)	mg/(8.h)
(ppt)	[pptr]	mg/(8.hr.kg)	mg/(8.h.kg)
(ppth)	[ppth]	mg/(kg.hr)	mg/(kg.h)
(th_u)	[todd'U]	mg/hr	mg/h
/(arb_u)	/[arb'U]	miu/mL	m[iU]/mL
/(hpf)	[HPF]	mL/((hb).m^2)	mL/{hb}.m^2
/(tot)	/{tot}	mL/(8.hr)	mL/(8.h)
/iu	/[iU]	mL/(8.hr.kg)	mL/(8.h.kg)
10*3(rbc)	10*3{rbc}	mL/(hb)	mL/{hb}
10.L	10.L/(min.m^2)	mL/(kg.hr)	mL/(kg.h)
10.un.s/(cm^5.m^2)	dyn.s/(cm^5.m^2)	mL/cm_h20	mL/cm[H20]
10.un.s/cm^5	dyn.s/cm^5	mL/hr	mL/h
cm_h20	cm[H20]	mm(hg)	mm[Hg]
cm_h20.s/L	cm[H20].s/L	mm/hr	mm/h
cm_h20/(s.m)	cm[H20]/(s.m)	mmol/(8.hr.kg)	mmol/(8.h.kg)
dba	dB[SPL]	mmol/(8hr)	mmol/(8h)

Table 17.4 (continued)

ISO+	UCUM	ISO+	UCUM
dm²/s²	REM	mmol/(kg.hr)	mmol/(kg.h)
g(creat)	g{creat}	mmol/hr	mmol/h
g(hgb)	g{hgb}	ng/(8.hr)	ng/(8.h)
g(tot_nit)	g{tit_nit}	ng/(8.hr.kg)	ng/(8.h.kg)
g(tot_prot)	g{tot_prot}	ng/(kg.hr)	ng/(kg.h)
g(wet_tis)	g{wet_tis}	ng/hr	ng/h
g.m/((hb).m2)	g.m/{hb}m²	osmol	osm
g.m/(hb)	g.m/{hb}	osmol/kg	osm/kg
g/(8.hr)	g/(8.h)	osmol/L	osm/L
g/(8.kg.hr)	g/(8.kg.h)	pa	pA
g/(kg.hr)	g/(kg.h)	pal	Pa
g/hr	g/h	sec	''
in	[in_us]	sie	S
in_hg	[in_i'Hg]	ug(8hr)	ug(8.h)
iu	[iU]	ug/(8.hr.kg)	ug/(8.h.kg)
iu/d	[iU]/d	ug/(kg.hr)	ug/(kg.h)
iu/hr	[iU]/h	ug/hr	ug/h
iu/kg	[iU]/kg	uiu	u[iU]

A great number of codes in ISO+ and UCUM are exactly the same (by design). These codes appear in the table below.

Table 17.5 Codes that are the same in ISO+ and UCUM

%	g/L	mg	ng/m²
/kg	g/m²	mg/(kg.d)	ng/min
/L	g/min	mg/(kg.min)	ng/mL
/m³	Gy	mg/d	ng/s
/min	H	mg/dL	nkat
/m³	hL	mg/kg	nm
/min	J/L	mg/L	nmol/s
/mL	kat	mg/m²	ns
1/mL	kat/kg	mg/m³	Ohm
10*12/L	kat/L	mg/min	Ohm.m

(continued)

Table 17.5 (continued)

10*3/L	kg	mL	pg
10*3/mL	kg.m/s	mL/(kg.d)	pg/L
10*3/mm³	kg/(s.m²)	mL/(kg.min)	pg/mL
10*6/L	kg/L	mL/(min.m²)	pkat
10*6/mL	kg/m³	mL/d	pm
10*6/mm³	kg/min	mL/kg	pmol
10*9/L	kg/mol	mL/m²	ps
10*9/mL	kg/s	mL/mbar	pt
10*9/mm³	kPa	mL/min	Sv
10.L/min	ks	mL/s	t
a/m	L	mm	ueq
bar	L.s	mmol/(kg.d)	ug
Bq	L/(min.m²)	mmol/(kg.min)	ug/(kg.d)
Cel	L/d	mmol/kg	ug/(kg.min)
cm	L/kg	mmol/L	ug/d
cm²/s	L/min	mmol/m²	ug/dL
d	L/s	mmol/min	ug/g
db	lm	mol/(kg.s)	ug/kg
deg	m	mol/kg	ug/L
eq	m/s²	mol/L	ug/m²
eV	m²	mol/m³	ug/min
f	m²/s	mol/s	ukat
fg	m³/s	mosm/L	um
fL	mbar	ms	umol
fmol	mbar.s/L	mv	umol/d
g	meq	n	umol/L
g.m	meq/(kg.d)	ng	umol/min
g/(kg.d)	meq/(kg.min)	ng/(kg.d)	us
g/(kg.min)	meq/d	ng/(kg.min)	uV
g/d	meq/kg	ng/d	V
g/dL	meq/L	ng/kg	Wb
g/kg	meq/min	ng/L	

Reference Range (OBX-7)

The reference range is given for numeric values in the form *lower-upper*, *<upper* or *>lower* as a string in this field. The units of the reference range are the same as the reported value (see OBX-6 above). When a reference range is given, it is included in the `<observation>` using the `<referenceRange>` element. An `<observationRange>` element should include a `<value>` using the IVL_PQ data type, where the unit is mapped from OBX-6, and the lower and upper bound are given in the `<low>` and `<high>` elements inside the `<value>`. When the lower or upper bound is omitted, the corresponding `<low>` or `<high>` element can simply be omitted. The `<interpretationCode>` of the `<observationRange>` should indicate that this range is for a normal interpretation. Note that CDA Release 2 also allows for reference ranges for abnormal results to be reported, but HL7 Version 2 only reports the normal range. The example below shows how one would report a reference range of 3.5-4.5 in CDA Release 2.0.

```
<referenceRange>
   <observationRange>
      <value xsi:type='IVL_PQ' unit='…'>
         <low value='3.5'/>
         <high value='4.5'/>
      </value>
      <observationInterpretation
         code='N' displayName='normal'
         codeSystem='2.16.840.1.113883.5.83'
         codeSystemName='ObservationInterpretation'
      />
   </observationRange>
</referenceRange>
```

Fig. 17.12 Reference Range Example

Abnormal Flags (OBX-8)

This field indicates whether the reported value is considered to be abnormal. The recommended CDA coding system is ObservationInterpretation and uses the same code values as are recommended by the HL7 Version 2 standard.

Probability (OBX-9)

When present this field indicates the likelihood of the value given. Its presence indicates a need for one of the probabilistic data types in HL7 Version 3, such as PPD<PQ>, UVN<CD> or UVP<CD>. These rarely appear in HL7 Version 2 messages.

Nature of Abnormal Test (OBX-10)

This field indicates how normal and abnormal values are determined (e.g., based on age, gender or race). It describes the type of `<referenceRange>` that is being produced, and so should appear in the `<code>` element of the `<observationRange>`.

Date/Time of Observation (OBX-14)

This field reports the date/time the observation was made. This value should be mapped to the `<effectiveTime>` element of the `<observation>` as the HL7 Version 2 standard describes this time as the physiologically relevant time (e.g., specimen collection time), not necessarily the time the actual value was determined or measured.

Producer ID (OBX-15)

This field represents the identifier of the producing service (e.g., an outside laboratory). It should be mapped into the `<id>` element of the `<assignedEntity>` of the `<performer>` associated with the `<observation>`.

Responsible Observer (OBX-16)

This field reports the person responsible for producing the result. The definition of this person in the HL7 Version 2 standard most closely matches the `<author>`. The identifier found in the first component should be mapped into the `<id>` of the `<assignedAuthor>` element. The name found in the second through eighth component should be mapped to the `<name>` element of the `<authorPerson>` element in the `<assignedAuthor>` element.

Observation Method (OBX-17)

This field reports more detail about the method of observation that is not captured in OBX-3. The `<methodCode>` element of the `<observation>` should be used to report the value of this field.

OBX Fields Not Mapped

The result status (OBX-11) addresses workflow for dynamic status reporting, and does not map into CDA which is a static document. Only preliminary, final or corrected results should be reported in a CDA document. To distinguish between these different types of results, one might use the `<methodCode>` of the `<observation>` or indicate through other means (e.g., presence or absence of an authenticator, or by referenced to a result being replaced) that a result has been verified or replaces a prior result. The OBX-12 field contains the date before which prior results using the same result code (OBX-3) would not be comparable due to changes in how normal values are computed. If CDA had allowed the `<observationRange>` to contain an `<effectiveTime>`, this would be the lower bound on it, but that RIM class attribute is not present on the `ObservationRange` class. OBX-13 is a rarely used field present to allow for receiver classification of results.

17.4
Transcription Document Header (TXA)

The TXA Segment has a great deal in common with information in the Clinical Document Header because this segment serves much the same purpose in HL7 Version 2 as the header of the clinical document. This segment is only used in document management messages (MDM), and is not present in other messages such as ADT or ORU messages. As a result, a number of key fields in a CDA document instance need to be filled in using proxies (substitutes) for the TXA fields.

Note that when a CDA is transmitted using an MDM message, Section 3 of the CDA standard recommends these same fields be filled in from the appropriate elements of the CDA document. The figure below shows where the fields in the TXA segment map to the CDA document header.

```
<ClinicalDocument>
    <id root='…' extension='TXA-12'/>
    <code code='TXA-2' codeSystem='2.16.840.1.113883.6.1'/>
    <effectiveTime value='TXA-6'/>
    <confidentialityCode code='TXA-18'
        codeSystem='2.16.840.1.113883.5.25'
        codeSystemName='Confidentiality' />
    <author>
        <time value='TXA-8'/>
        <assignedAuthor>
            <id root='…' extension='TXA-9.1'/>
            <authorPerson>
                <name>TXA-9.2 - TXA-9.8</name>
            </authorPerson>
        </assignedAuthor>
    </author>
    <legalAuthenticator>
        <signatureCode code='I'/>
        <assignedEntity>
            <id root='…' extension='TXA-10.1'/>
            <assignedPerson>
                <name>TXA-10.2 - TXA-10.8</name>
            </assignedPerson>
        </assignedEntity>
    </legalAuthenticator>
    <legalAuthenticator>
        <time value='TXA-22.15'/>
        <signatureCode code='S'/>
```

Fig. 17.13 TXA to CDA ClinicalDocument mapping

```
        <assignedEntity>
            <id root='…' extension='TXA-22.1'/>
            <assignedPerson>
                <name>TXA-22.2 - TXA-22.8</name>
            </assignedPerson>
        </assignedEntity>
    </legalAuthenticator>
    <intendedRecipient>
        <informationRecipient>
            <id root='…' extension='TXA-23.1'/>
            <intendedRecipient>
                <name>TXA-23.2 - TXA-23.8</name>
            </intendedRecipient>
        </informationRecipient>
    </intendedRecipient>
    <dataEnterer>
        <time value='TXA-7'/>
        <assignedEntity>
            <id root='…' extension='TXA-11.1'/>
            <assignedPerson>
                <name>TXA-11.2 - TXA-11.8</name>
            </assignedPerson>
        </assignedEntity>
    </dataEnterer>
    <relatedDocument typeCode='EVN-2'>
        <parentDocument>
            <id root='…' extension='TXA-13'/>
        </parentDocument>
    </relatedDocument>
    <documentationOf>
        <serviceEvent>
            <effectiveTime value='TXA-4'/>
            <performer>
                <assignedEntity>
                    <id root='…' extension='TXA-5.1'/>
                    <assignedPerson>
                        <name>TXA-5.2 - TXA-5.8</name>
                    </assignedPerson>
                </assignedEntity>
            </performer>
        </serviceEvent>
    </documentationOf>
    <infulfillmentOf>
        <order>
            <id root='…' extension='TXA-14'/>
            <id root='…' extension='TXA-15'/>
        </order>
    </infulfillmentOf>
</ClinicalDocument>
```

Fig. 17.13 (continued)

Document Type (TXA-2)

The Document Type field in TXA-2 should be mapped into an appropriate LOINC code and placed in the `<code>` element of the `<ClinicalDocument>`.

Activity Date/Time (TXA-4)

TXA-4 describes the date/time of the activity (the service event) describe in the document. This should appear in the `<effectiveTime>` element of the `<serviceEvent>` in the CDA instance.

Primary Activity Provider (TXA-5)

The primary activity provider is the performer of the service event and should be recorded in the `<performer>` element of the `<serviceEvent>` in the CDA instance.

Origination Date/Time (TXA-6)

The time that the document was created is stored in the `<effectiveTime>` element of the `<ClinicalDocument>`.

Transcription Date/Time (TXA-7)

The time of transcription should be stored in the `<time>` element of the `<dataEnterer>`. It may also be used as a proxy for the TXA-6 when neither TXA-6 nor TXA-8 fields are present.

Edit Date/Time (TXA-8)

This field contains the date/time stamp for when the document was edited. For an original document notification, this is often the same as the document creation time, and when TXA-6 is missing, this field can serve as a proxy for it. It can also be used as a proxy for the `<time>` element in the `<author>`.

Originator (TXA-9)

Field TXA-9 can contain both the name and identifier of the document author. The identifier is the first component of TXA-9 and should be placed in the `<id>` element of the `<author>` in the CDA instance. Components 2 through 8 of this field should be placed in the `<name>` element of the `<assignedPerson>` element in the `<author>`.

Assigned Document Authenticator (TXA-10)

This field is intended to record the person from whom a signature is required. This records an authenticator where the `code` XML attribute of the `<signatureCode>` element is set to the value X indicating that a signature is required or expected of this person. Note that this field differs from TXA-22 which indicates that a signature has been provided.

When TXA-10 is present, its contents should appear in either the `<legalAuthen-ticator>` or `<authenticator>` elements of the CDA instance. The element used should be based on the organizational policy for filling in TXA-22. If this field is completed with the expected legal signer of the document, then it should appear in `<legal-Authenticator>`, otherwise it should appear in the `<authenticator>` element. The first component of TXA-10 contains the authenticators ID and should appear in the `<id>` element of the `<assignedEntity>` appearing in the chosen element. Again, components 2 through 8 are the authenticator's name and should appear in the `<name>` element of the `<assignedPerson>`.

Transcriptioninst (TXA-11)

This field contains the name (components 2 through 8) and identifier (component 1) of the person who transcribed the document. This information is captured in the `<dataEn-terer>` element in the CDA instance. The name is placed in the `<name>` element of the `<assignedPerson>`. If present the identifier should appear in the `<id>` element of the `<assignedEntity>` for the `<dataEnterer>`.

Unique Document Number (TXA-12)

This field uniquely identifies the document and should be placed in the `<id>` element of the `<ClinicalDocument>`.

Parent Document Number (TXA-13)

This field appears when documents are addended (T05 or T06) or replaced (T09 and T10). The event (addendum or replacement) is indicated in the `<typeCode>` element beneath the `<relatedDocument>`. The parent document identifier is placed in the `<id>` element of the `<parentDocument>`. The value of the `typeCode` XML attribute on the `<relatedDocument>` should be mapped from the event type recorded in the EVN segment.

Placer (TXA-14) and Filler (TXA-15) Order Numbers

These fields identify relevant order numbers that are fulfilled by the document. The order numbers should appear in `extension` XML attribute of the `<id>` element of the `<order>` element in the `<infulfillmentOf>` in the CDA instance. The `root` attribute of the <id> element should contain the appropriate OID to identify whether the source of the identifier is the order placer or order filler.

Document Completion Status (TXA-17)

This field indicates the current status of the document. When it contains a value of AU it means that the document is signed, and when it contains a value of LA it means that the document is legally authenticated. It can be used to determine whether the signer found in TXA-22 should be stored in the <authenticator> or <legalAuthenticator> element.

Document Confidentiality Status (TXA-18)

This field uses nearly the same set of codes as the CDA standard. The three values are U (Usual Control), R (Restricted) and V (Very Restricted). CDA recommends a vocabulary using the codes N, R and V to mean the same things respectively. This field would appear in the <confidentialityCode> element of the <ClinicalDocument>.

Authentication Person and Time Stamp (TXA-22)

This field is made up of several components. The first part identifies the authenticating person, the second through eighth give the authenticator's name, and the fifteenth indicates the time at which the document was authenticated (signed). Depending on the type of authentication (see TXA-17) this contents of this field should be placed in either the <legalAuthenticator> or the <authenticator> element. When TXA-17 is not valued, where the information goes needs to be determined by the organizational policies for how documents are signed. The identifier in component 1 goes in the <id> element under the <assignedEntity> in the chosen element. The name found in components 2 through 8 go into the <name> element of the <assignedPerson> under the <assignedEntity> element. The time of authentication found in component 15 should go into the <time> element of the chosen <authenticator> or <legalAu-thenticator> element. If the time is not specified in component 15, then EVN-2 (event time) or MSH-7 (message time) may be used as a proxy for the signature time based on organizational policy.

Distributed Copies (TXA-23)

This field identifies the people who have received or are to receive copies of the document. Again, the identifier is found in the first component and the name of the person receiving copies is found in components 2 through 8. The identifier should be stored in the <id> element of the <intendedRecipient> and the name in the <name> element found in the <informationRecpient> under the <intendedRecipient> element.

Unmapped Fields in the TXA Segment

TXA-1 is the Set ID and simply serves to identify the TXA segment for workflow. TXA-3 indicates how the document was created and is not present in the CDA header. TXA-16 gives a file name for the document and is not used in the CDA header. TXA-19 through TXA-21 are used to control workflow and represent document status changes. A CDA document is not altered during status changes, so these fields do not apply "inside" the document. They would instead control workflow operations such as deprecation or removal of a deleted document.

17.5
Patient Identifier (PID)

The PID segment maps onto the <recordTarget> participation. The figure below shows where the fields of the PID segment appear in that element.

```
<recordTarget>
    <patientRole>
        <id root='…' extension='PID-2,3,4,18,19,20'/>
        <addr>PID-11
            <county>PID-12</county>
        </addr>
        <telecom value='PID-13' use='H'/>
        <telecom value='PID-14' use='W'/>
        <patient>
            <name>PID-5</name><name use='P'>PID-9</name>
            <administrativeGenderCode code='PID-8' …/>
            <birthTime value='PID-7' … />
            <maritalStatusCode code='PID-16' …/>
            <religiousAffiliationCode code='PID-17' …/>
            <raceCode code='PID-10' …/>
            <ethnicGroupCode code='PID-22' …/>
            <birthPlace>
                <place>
                        <name>PID-23</name>
                        <addr>PID-23</addr>
                </place>
            </birthPlace>
            <languageCommunication>
                    <languageCode code='PID-15'/>
                </languageCommunication>
        </patient>
    </patientRole>
</recordTarget>
```

Fig. 17.14 PID to CDA recordTarget mapping

Patient ID (PID-2), Patient ID List (PID-3) and Alternate ID (PID-4)

These four fields all represent some sort of patient identity. Some applications use PID-2, others PID-2 and PID-4, and others only PID-3. Values in these fields should be mapped to the <id> element of the <patientRole> found in the <recordTarget>.

Patient Name (PID-5)

This field supplies the patient name as should be mapped to the <name> element of the <patient> found in the <patientRole> element.

Mother's Maiden Name (PID-6)

The mother's maiden name appears in the PID segment to help distinguish between patients with the same given and family name. However, in CDA Release 2.0, there is no appropriate place beneath <recordTarget> where this information would appear. Instead, a <participant> would need to be added to the CDA header that identified the mother of the patient.

```
<participant typeCode='IND'>
   <associatedEntity classCode='PRS'>
       <id root='…' extension='…'/>
       <code code='MTHR' codeSystem=''/>
       <associatedPerson>
           <name>
               <family qualifier='BR'>Maiden Name</family>
           </name>
       </associatedPerson>
   </associatedEntity>
</participant>
```

Fig. 17.15 Representing the mother's maiden name

Date/Time of Birth (PID-7)

This field is mapped to the <birthTime> element of the <patient> element.

Sex (PID-8)

This field is mapped to the <administrativeGenderCode> element of the <patient> element.

Patient Alias (PID-9)

This field supplies an alternate patient name and should also be mapped to the <name> element of the <patient> found in the <patientRole> element. The use XML attribute of the <name> should contain an appropriate value (e.g., P for a pseudonym) to indicate that this is some type of alternative name.

Race (PID-10)

This field is mapped to the <raceCode> element of the <patient> element.

Patient Address (PID-11)

This field is mapped to the <addr> element of the <patientRole> element.

County (PID-12)

This field is mapped to a <county> element found in the <addr> element of the <patientRole> element.

Phone Number – Home (PID-13) and – Business (PID-14)

PID-13 and PID-14 use the HL7 Version 2 XTN data type. Although component 1 is included for backwards compatibility and the HL7 Version 2.3.1 standard recommends use of components 5 through 8 to represent the parsed phone number, most implementations still use the first component for the phone number. The first component of this field is mapped to the value attribute of a <telecom> element in the <patientRole> element. The telephone number needs to be translated into the tel: URL format defined in RFC 3966. The second component of this field indicates the use of the phone number, and can be mapped to the use XML attribute in the <telecom> element. Typically this field is NOT present since PID-13 is described as being the home phone number and PID-14 is the business phone number.

```
<telecom use='HP' value='tel:+14844362322'/>
```

Fig. 17.16 Telephone number mapping

The fourth component if present is an e-mail address and would be mapped to an additional <telecom> element.

```
<telecom use='HP' value='mailto:name@anydomain'/>
```

Fig. 17.17 e-Mail address mapping

Primary Language (PID-15)

This field is mapped to the `<languageCode>` element found in `<languageCommu-nication>` appearing in the `<patient>` element.

Marital Status (PID-16)

This field is mapped to the `<maritalStatusCode>` element of the `<patient>` element.

Religion (PID-17)

This field is mapped to the `<religiousAffiliationCode>` element of the `<patient>` element.

Patient Account Number (PID-18), SSN Number (PID-19) and Driver's License Number (PID-20)

These fields are just other kinds of patient identifiers and may be placed in the `<id>` element of the `<patientRole>`.

Mother's Identifier (PID-21)

This field should be mapped to the `<id>` element shown in the `<participant>` in Fig. 17.15 above.

Ethnic Group (PID-22)

This field is mapped to the `<ethnicGroupCode>` element of the `<patient>` element.

Birth Place (PID-23)

This field indicates the place of birth of the patient. It can indicate a political boundary (county, state or country) or the name of a place (e.g., a hospital) where the patient was born. This is stored in the `<place>` element appearing inside `<birthPlace>` of the `<patient>` element. If the birthplace is a political boundary, the `<addr>` element of the `<place>` would contain `<county>`, `<state>` or `<country>` element as appropriate. If the place is just the name of a location, then it can be mapped to the `<name>` of the `<place>`.

Fields Not Mapped

Multiple Birth Indicator (PID-24) and Birth Order (PID-25) are used to distinguish between different children of multiple births (who may not yet be named). There is no place in the `<recordTarget>` to place this information, but they could be mapped into the `<value>` elements of `<observation>` elements that represented the appropriate concepts.

The Citizenship (PID-26), Veterans Military Status (PID-27), Nationality (PID-28), Patient Death Date and Time (PID-29), Patient Death Indicator (PID-30) provide more demographic data about the patient. These would also need to be mapped into the `<value>` elements of `<observation>` elements that represented the appropriate concepts.

17.6
Patient Visit Information (PV1)

The PV1 segment is used to communicate information about the visit. In the CDA standard, this information would appear in the `<encompassingEncounter>` element in the CDA Header.

```
<encompassingEncounter>
    <id root='…' extension='PV1-19'/>
    <id root='…' extension='PV1-5' />
    <id root='…' extension='PV1-50' />
    <code code='PV1-2+PV1-10'/>
    <effectiveTime>
    <low value='PV1-44'/><high value='PV1-45'/>
    </effectiveTime>
    <dischargeDispositionCode code='PV1-36' …/>
    <location>
        <healthCareFacility>
            <id extension='PV1-39'/>
            <code code=''/>
            <encounterParticipant typeCode='PV1-7,8,9,17'>
                <assignedEntity>
                    <id root='…'
                        extension='PV1-7.1,8.1,9.1,17.1'/>
```

Fig. 17.18 PV1 to CDA encompassingEncounter mapping

```
            <assignedPerson>
                <name>(PV1-7,8,9,17).2-7</name>
            </assignedPerson>
        </assignedEntity>
    </encounterParticipant>
    <location>
        <name>PV1-3</name>
        <addr></addr>
    </location>
  </healthCareFacility>
 </location>
</encompassingEncounter>
```

Fig 17.18 (continued)

Patient Class (PV1-2)

This field can be mapped to the `<code>` element in `<encompassingEncounter>` to indicate the type of visit. See also Hospital Service (PV1-10) below.

Assigned Patient Location (PV1-3)

This field can be mapped into the `<name>` element found in the `<location>` under the `<healthcareFacility>` element of the `<encompassingEncounter>`.

Preadmit Number (PV1-5)

This field is the preadmission account number. It may be used as an identifier for the visit, in which case it should appear in the `<id>` element of the `<encompassing Encounter>`.

Attending Doctor (PV1-7), Referring Doctor (PV1-8), Consulting Doctor (PV1-9) and Admitting Doctor (PV1-17)

These fields identify different participants in the encounter, and so appear beneath `<encounterParticipant>` elements. Component 1 should appear in the `<id>` element of the `<assignedEntity>` in the `<encounterParticipant>`. Component s 2 through 7 should appear in the `<name>` element of the `<assignedPerson>` element in the `<assignedEntity>`. The typeCode XML attribute of the `<encounterParticipant>` element should be set to ATND, REF, CON or ADM for attending, referring, consulting or admitting; depending upon whether the information is found in PV1-7, PV1-8, PV1-9 or PV1-17 respectively.

Hospital Service (PV1-10)

This field can be mapped to the `<code>` element in `<encompassingEncounter>` to indicate the type of visit. See also Patient Class (PV1-2) above.

VIP Indicator (PV1-16)

Contents of this field might be used to inform the value selected for `<confidentialityCode>` in the `<ClinicalDocument>`.

Visit Number (PV1-19)

This field should appear in the `<id>` element of the `<encompassingEncounter>`.

Discharge Disposition (PV1-36)

This field should be mapped to the `<dischargeDispositionCode>` element of the `<encompassingEncounter>`.

Servicing Facility (PV1-39)

This field should be mapped to the `<id>` element of the `<healthCareFacility>` element found in the `<encompassingEncounter>`.

Admit Date/Time (PV1-44)

This field should be mapped to the `<low>` element of the `<effectiveTime>` found in the `<encompassingEncounter>`. It may also be mapped to the same element in a `<serviceEvent>` that represents the encounter.

Discharge Date/Time (PV1-45)

This field should be mapped to the `<high>` element of the `<effectiveTime>` found in the `<encompassingEncounter>`. It may also be mapped to the same element in a `<serviceEvent>` that represents the encounter.

Alternate Visit ID (PV1-50)

This field should appear in the `<id>` element of the `<encompassingEncounter>`.

Other Healthcare Provider (PV1-52)

This field is very similar in structure to PV1-7, PV1-8, PV1-9 and PV1-17. It identifies other participants in the encounter, and so would be expected to appear as an encounter participant. However, the CDA standard limits these to just a small set of values. The best place to put these participants is in `<performer>` of a `<serviceEvent>` related to this encounter, or as a `<participant>` in the CDA Header. The typeCode XML attribute and contents of the `<code>` and `<functionCode>` elements would need to be determined by local policy.

Unmapped Fields

Numerous fields are not mapped because they apply to billing rather than documentation of the encounter. Other fields address bed management, referral workflows, or visit accommodations.

17.7
Additional Patient Visit Information (PV2)

The PV2 segment contains additional information about the visit. Most of this is not mapped to the CDA document in any uniform way. However, the Admit Reason (PV2-3) and Transfer Reason (PV2-4) fields could appear in a "Reason for Visit" section (LOINC 29299-5) in the body of the CDA document.

17.8
Next of Kin (NK1)

This segment maps to <participant> elements in the <ClinicalDocument> as it describes next of kin, emergency contacts, employer or school contacts. Usually the typeCode XML attribute on the <participant> element should be set to IND to indicate that they are an indirect participant in the encounter.

```
<participant typeCode='IND'>
   <time>
      <low value='NK1-8'/><high value='NK1-9'/>
   </time>
   <associatedEntity classCode='NK1-7'>
      <id root='…' extension='NK1-12,33,37'/>
      <code code='NK1-3+NK1-7' …/>
      <addr>NK1-4</addr>
      <telecom value='NK1-4' use='H'/>
      <telecom value='NK1-5' use='W'/>
      <associatedPerson>
         <name>NK1-2</name>
      </associatedPerson>
      <scopingOrganization>
         <name>NK1-13</name>
      </scopingOrganization>
   </associatedEntity>
</participant>
```

Fig. 17.19 NK1 to CDA participant mapping

Name (NK1-2)

Components 1 through 6 of this field can be mapped to the <name> element of the <associatedPerson> in the <associatedEntity> element of the <participant>.

Relationship (NK1-3)

This field identifies the type of relationship between the person described in the NK1 segment and the patient. The values used in this field usually affects the <code> element and should be mapped to values from the HL7 PersonalRelationshipRoleType value set found in the HL7 Role Code Vocabulary. It may sometimes affect the classCode XML attribute of the <assignedEntity> element as well (see Role NK1-7 below).

Address (NK1-4)

This field should be mapped to the <addr> element in the <associatedEntity> element appearing in the <participant>.

Phone Number (NK1-5)

This field should be mapped to the `<telecom>` element in the `<associatedEntity>` element appearing in the `<participant>`. The use XML attribute of the `<telecom>` element should be set to H.

Business Phone Number (NK1-6)

This field should be mapped to the `<telecom>` element in the `<associatedEntity>` element appearing in the `<participant>`. The use XML attribute of the `<telecom>` element should be set to W.

Contact Role (NK1-7)

This field identifies the role of the contact person. It influences the value that should appear in the XML classCode attribute of the `<associatedEntity>` in the `<participant>` element.

Description	classCode
Someone acting as an agent patient.	AGNT
The person responsible for the patient's care at home.	CAREGIVER
A contact person for an employer, school or other agency related to the patient.	CON
An emergency contact for the patient.	ECON
The patient's designated next-of-kin.	NOK
Someone in a personal relationship with the patient.	PRS
The patient's guardian	GUARD[a]

[a]Guardians must appear in the `<guardian>` element under the `<patient>` rather than as a separate `<participant>` element.

When an employer, school or other contact is included, the `<code>` element of the `<associatedEntity>` can be used to distinguish between different varieties of contacts. The IHE PCC Technical Framework defines three codes for contacts to augment HL7 Vocabularies for role. This is a subset of the IHE RoleCode vocabulary, which has the identifier 1.3.5.1.4.1.19376.1.5.3.3

These or other similar codes can be used to further distinguish relationships in the `<code>` element.

Code	Meaning
EMPLOYER	The employer of a person.
SCHOOL	The school in which a person is enrolled.
AFFILIATED	An organization with which a person is affiliated (e.g., a volunteer organization).

Start Date (NK1-8) and End Date (NK1-9)

These fields indicate the start and end date of the relationship between the contact and the patient. They can be mapped into the <low> and <high> elements of the <time> in the <participant> element.

Organization Name – NK1 (NK1-13)

This field can be mapped to the <name> element of the <scopingOrganization> inside the <associatedEntity> element.

Next of Kin/Associated Parties Employee Number (NK1-12), Next of Kin/Associated Party's Identifiers (NK1-33), and Contact Person Social Security Number (NK1-37)

These fields can serve as identifiers for the contact, and so would appear in the <id> element of the <associatedEntity>.

Fields Not Mapped

Most of the fields in NK1 that have not been mapped contain more demographic detail about the person reported in the NK1 segment, including gender, date of birth, et cetera. There is no place for this level of demographic detail in the CDA Release 2 standard.

17.9
Message Header (MSH) and Event (EVN) Segments

Sending Facility (MSH-4)

This field identifies the sending facility. The contents of this field can be used to locate the correct values to fill in for a number of the scoping organization elements in the CDA Header, including <representedOrganization> for the <author>, <authenticator> and <legalAuthenticator> elements. It can also be used to fill in values for the <representedCustodianOrganization> element of the <assignedCustodian> element.

Message Date/Time (MSH-7)

The date and time of the message is often used a proxy for other document related events. When CDA documents are transformed from messages, the message date / time is often used as the document creation time and appears in the `<effectiveTime>` element of the `<ClinicalDocument>` element. The message date/time can also be used to help create a unique id for the document (but see also MSH-10).

Message Control Id (MSH-10)

This is the unique identifier for the message being sent. This value is often used to create a unique identifier for the clinical document stored in the `<id>` element of the `<ClinicalDocument>` element.

Recorded Date/Time (EVN-2) and Occurred Date/Time (EVN-6)

These fields record the time that the event was recorded and the time that it actually occurred (it could have be recorded after it occurred). Either of these dates can also serve as a proxy for document related events such as the document creation time (see MSH-7 above).

17.10
Common Order Segment (ORC)

The ORC segment was developed to report information common to orders, and is used in a number of ordering related messages. This segment sometimes appears in ORU messages that represent responses (e.g., results) for an ordered test.

```
<infulfillmentOf>
   <order>
           <id root='…' extension='ORC-2'/>
           <id root='…' extension='ORC-3'/>
           <id root='…' extension='ORC-4'/>
           <id root='…' extension='ORC-8'/>
   </order>
</infulfillmentOf>
<encounterParticipant typeCode='REF'>
   <assignedEntity>
           <id root='…' extension='ORC-12.1'/>
           <addr>ORC-24</addr>
           <telecom value='ORC-14'/>
```

Fig. 17.20 ORC mapping to infulfillmentOf

```
            <assignedPerson>
                <name>ORC-12.2-7</name>
            </assignedPerson>
            <representedOrganization>
                    <id root='…' extension='ORC-12.1'/>
                    <name>ORC-21</name>
                    <telecom value='ORC-23'>
                    <addr>ORC-22</addr>
            </representedOrganization>
        </assignedEntity>
</encounterParticipant>
```

Fig 17.20 (continued)

Placer Order Number (ORC-2) and Filler Order Number (ORC-3)

These fields represent order numbers associated with the message. When the message is reporting results of an order, these fields should be mapped to the <id> elements of the <order> found in the <infulfillmentOf> element of the CDA header.

Placer Group Number (ORC-4)

This field identifies a group of orders, and can appear in the same location as the placer order number (ORC-2) or filler order number (ORC-3) in the CDA document. This indicates that the CDA document fulfills part of the order group.

Order Status (ORC-5)

This field is not typically mapped into the CDA document, but its values can be used to determine whether or not a document might need to be created in response to an ORU message. Some ORU messages might simply be reporting that an order is in process or has been cancelled, and it would make no sense to produce a document for these events.

Parent (ORC-8)

This field when present indicates the parent order. Again, its contents can be mapped into the <order> element.

Ordering Provider (ORC-12)

This field can be mapped to an <encounterParticipant> in the CDA Header. The typeCode XML attribute on that element should be REF to indicate that this is the physician who referred the patient for these services (e.g., ordered the test). Component 1 of ORC-12 would appear in the `<id>` element of the `<assignedEntity>` in the `<encounterParticipant>` element. Components 2 through 8 would appear in the `<name>` element of the `<assignedPerson>` found in the `<assignedEntity>`.

Callback Phone Number (ORC-14)

This field can be mapped to the `<telecom>` element of the `<assignedEntity>` used for the Ordering Provider (ORC-12) above.

Ordering Facility Name (ORC-21)

This field can be mapped to the `<name>` element of the `<representedOrganization>` in the `<assignedEntity>` of the `<encounterParticipant>` described above for Ordering Provider (ORC-12).

Ordering Facility Address (ORC-22)

This field can be mapped to the `<addr>` element of the `<representedOrganization>` in the `<assignedEntity>` of the `<encounterParticipant>` described above for Ordering Provider (ORC-12).

Ordering Facility Phone Number (ORC-23)

This field can be mapped to the `<telecom>` element of the `<representedOrganization>` in the `<assignedEntity>` of the `<encounterParticipant>` described above for Ordering Provider (ORC-12).

Ordering Provider Address (ORC-24)

This field can be mapped to the `<addr>` element of the of the `<assignedEntity>` of the `<encounterParticipant>` described above for Ordering Provider (ORC-12).

17.11
Observation Request Segment (OBR)

The OBR segment represents an order request. As such, it most accurately would be represented in an `<observation>` element where the moodCode XML attribute is set to RQO. However an ORU message can often contain a number of these, and they also make good places to insert `<section>` elements in the CDA document. If you use them as `<section>` elements, you should report the OBX segments under the OBR in the `<section>` that the OBR was mapped to.

```
<organizer>
   <effectiveTime value='OBR-7'><!-- if OBR-8 is empty -->
       <low value='OBR-7'/>
       <high value='OBR-8'/>
   </effectiveTime>
   <component>
       <!-- information about the order -->
   <observation moodCode='RQO'>
           <id root='…' extension='OBR-2,3'/>
           <priorityCode code='OBR-5'/>
           <code code='OBR-4.1' …>
               <translation code='OBR-4.2'/>
           </code>
           <priorityCode code='OBR-5' …/>
           <entryRelationship typeCode='RSON'>
               <observation moodCode='EVN'>
                   <code code='…'/>
                   <value xsi:type='CD' code='OBR-31'/>
               </observation>
           </entryRelationship>
           <author>
               <time value='OBR-6'/>
               <assignedAuthor>
                   <id extension='OBR-16.1'/>
                   <addr></addr>
                   <telecom value='OBR-17'/>
                   <assignedPerson>
                       <name>OBR-16.2-8</name>
                   </assignedPerson>
               </assignedAuthor>
           </author>
       </observation>
   </component>
   <component>
       <!-- information about the specimen -->
       <procedure>
           <targetSiteCode code='OBR-15.2' …/>
           <performer>
               <assignedEntity root='…'
                   extension='OBR-10.1'/>
                   <assignedPerson>
                       <name>OBR-10.2 through 10.8<name>
                   </assignedPerson>
               </assignedEntity>
           </performer>
           <specimen>
               <specimenRole>
                   <specimenPlayingEntity>
                       <code code='OBR-15.1' …/>
                       <quantity value='OBR-9.1'
                                 unit='OBR-9.2'/>
```

Fig. 17.21 OBR to CDA observation mapping

```
                  </specimenPlayingEntity>
               </specimenRole>
            </specimen>
         </procedure>
   </component>
<!-- one of these components should appear for
      every OBX beneath the OBR. -->
 <component>
    <observation moodCode='EVN'>
    </observation>
    </component>
</organizer>
```

Fig 17.21 (continued)

```
<component>
   <section>
      <code code='OBR-4' .../>
      <text></text>
      <author>
         <assignedAuthor>
            <id extension='OBR-32.1'/>
            <assignedPerson>
               <name>OBR-32.2-8</name>
            </assignedPerson>
         </assignedAuthor>
      </author>
      <entry>
         <organizer>See above</organizer>
      </entry>
   </section>
</component>
```

Fig. 17.22 OBR to CDA section mapping

Placer Order Number (OBR-2) and Filler Order Number (OBR-3)

These fields can be reported in the `<id>` element of the `<observation>` associated with the OBR to identify the request.

Universal Service ID (OBR-4)

This field contains the code for the service (the observation) that was requested. It should go into the `<code>` element of the `<observation>`, and if an OBR is mapped to a `<section>` element, the `<code>` element in the `<section>`. An alternate service ID, if present, should be placed in the `<translation>` element under the `<code>` described above.

Priority (OBR-5)

This field can be mapped to the `<priorityCode>` element of the `<observation>` for associated with the OBR segment.

Requested Date/Time (OBR-6)

The requested date and time of the order should be mapped to the `<time>` element for the `<author>` participant associated with the order. Note, this is not an ideal mapping, but CDA does not support the appropriate RIM classes or attributes to support an ideal mapping.

Observation Date/Time (OBR-7), Observation End Date/Time (OBR-8)

These field should be mapped to the `<low>` and `<high>` components of the `<effectiveTime>` in the `<observation>` elements that the OBX elements beneath the OBR are mapped to. It can also be mapped to the `<effectiveTime>` used in the `<organizer>` that groups them together.

Collection Volume (OBR-9)

This field should be mapped to the `<quantity>` element in the `<specimenPlayingEntity>`.

Collector ID (OBR-10)

This field identifies the performer of the specimen collection procedure. Component 1 of this field would be mapped to the `<id>` of the `<assignedEntity>` found in a `<performer>` element on the `<procedure>` element that reported the specimen collection activity. Components 2 through 8 would be recorded in the `<name>` element of the `<assignedPerson>` in the `<assignedEntity>`.

Relevant Clinical Information (OBR-13)

This would appear as a simple piece of text associated with the order request. See NTE below.

Specimen Source (OBR-15)

This field identifies the source of the specimen. The first component identifies the kind of specimen collected and should be mapped into the `<code>` element of the `<specimenPlayingEntity>` Component four of this field identifies the body site, and can be mapped into the `<targetSiteCode>` element of the specimen collection `<procedure>`.

Ordering Provider (OBR-16)

This field is exactly the same as Ordering Provider ORC-12. See that section above for details.

Order Callback Phone Number (OBR-17)

This field is exactly the same as Callback Phone Number ORC-13. See that section above for details.

Placer Field 1 (OBR-18)

While HL7 uses this as an open field, it is commonly used to record the Accession Number of the study associated with an imaging order. An imaging study is itself is a rather large observation, and so this field could be viewed as the identifier for that observation.

Diagnostic Serv Sect ID (OBR-24)

This field describes the location where the service (the result) was performed or produced. It could be mapped to the `<code>` in the `<healthcareFacility>`.

Result Status (OBR-25)

This field is not typically mapped into the CDA document, but its values can be used to determine whether or not a document might need to be created in response to an ORU message. Some ORU messages might simply be reporting that an order is in process or has been cancelled, and it would make no sense to produce a document for these events.

Parent Result (OBR-26)

This field identifies the observation upon which this request is being performed. For example, in microbial sensitivity, the observation reporting the microbe is the subject of a secondary observation about that microbe's sensitivity to particular treatments.

This field maps to the `<id>` of the parent observation. To record the linkage between the two:

```
<observation moodCode='RQO'><!-- Observation requested -->
   <entryRelationship typeCode='SUBJ'>
      <id …/> <!-- filled in from OBR-26 -->
      <code nullFlavor='UNK'/>
   </entryRelationship>
</observation>
```

Fig. 17.23 Parent result mapping

Result Copies to (OBR-28)

This field should be mapped to the `<informationRecipient>` element in the CDA Header. The first component maps to the `<id>` element of the `<intendedRecipient>` element in the `<informationRecipient>`. The second through eighth component can be mapped to `<name>` element of the `<informationRecipient>` element in the `<intendedRecipient>`.

```
<informationRecipient>
   <intendedRecipient>
      <id …/> <!-- filled in from OBR-28.1 -->
      <informationRecipient>
         <name>
            <!-- filled in from OBR-28.2 through 8 -->
         </name>
      </informationRecipient>
   </intendedRecipient>
</informationRecipient>
```

Parent (OBR-29)

This field is identical to Parent in ORC-8 above.

Reason for Study (OBR-31)

The reason for the study can be mapped into an `<observation>` that is associated with the `<observation>` used for most of the OBR using an `<entryRelationship>` element where the typeCode XML attribute is RSON.

Principal Result Interpreter (OBR-32) and Assistant Result Interpreter (OBR-33)

The interpreter is the person who authored the observations found in the OBX segments beneath the OBR, and can be placed in an `<author>` element in the `<section>`

where these are recorded. The <id> element of the <assignedAuthor> should come from the first component of the field. The <name> element in the <authorPerson> should contain the name found in the second through eighth component of the field.

17.12
Note (NTE)

The contents of the NTE segment represent a comment. When mapped to a CCD comment, this will always be <act> and the <code> element in it will use LOINC code 48767-8 Annotation comment. In a few other cases, this could also be mapped to <observation> and I would recommend use of the same <code> value. As a generate rule of thumb, if a document uses other CCD structures, then it should use the CCD <act> form for comments also.

Comments should appear in the elements that they are associated with using the subject <entryRelationship>. Because the subject relationship "arrow" goes in the direction opposite the nesting, you must set the inversionInd XML attribute to true. This is shown in the example below.

```
<entryRelationship typeCode='SUBJ' inversionInd='true'>
    <act classCode='ACT' moodCode='EVN'>
        <code code='48767-8'
            displayName='Annotation Comment'
            codeSystem='2.16.840.1.113883.6.1'
            codeSystemName='LOINC'/>
        <text>TEXT OF COMMENT</text>
        <author>
            ...
        </author>
    </act>
</entryRelationship>
```

Fig. 17.24 NTE to CDA comment example

Other types annotations (see Comment Type below) would be mapped to similar structures, but may use INT for the moodCode XML attribute value.

Source of Comment (NTE-2)

This is simply an identifier that indicates which participant was the source of the comment. The HL7 table for this field has three values to distinguish between comments from the filler, placer or other commenter, but this table can be extended. This field might be used to help identify the <author> associated with the comment.

Comment (NTE-3)

This field contains the comment that was made and will appear in the `<text>` element of the `<act>` (or `<observation>`) element containing the comment.

Comment Type (NTE-4)

Comments are of various forms. The HL7 Version 2 table 364 includes types for patient instructions, ancillary instructions, general instructions, primary and secondary reason, general reason, remark and duplicate/interaction reason.

Only comments of type remark should really be mapped to the CCD comment form. Other comment types, such as instructions should be mapped to similar structures but use a different code.

The IHE Patient Care Coordination Technical Framework supplies codes for Patient Instructions (PINSTRUCT) and Fulfillment Instructions (FINSTRUCT) and XML templates for those types of annotations.

The various "reason" codes would indicate that the relationship being represented is no longer an annotation on a subject, but the reason for a particular service. In these cases, the `<entryRelationship>` is written as shown in the figure below. Note the absence of the inversionInd flag in this example.

```
<entryRelationship typeCode='RSON'>
```

Fig. 17.25 Reasons

17.13
Specimens (SPM)

The SPM segment was introduced in HL7 Version 2.5 to support better reporting of specimen information. It maps to the `<specimen>` participation in the CDA model. The specimen is produced by a specimen collection procedure, and so appears inside a `<procedure>` element. The `<procedure>` element tracks details about how the specimen was collected.

```
<procedure>
   <code code='SPM-7' …/>
   <effectiveTime value='SPM-17'/>
   <approachSiteCode code='SPM-10' … />
   <targetSiteCode code='SPM-8' … >
      <qualifier>
         <name nullFlavor='NA'>
            <originalText
               >Modifier</originalText></name>
         <value code='SPM-9' … />
      </qualifier>
   </targetSiteCode>
   <specimen>
      <specimenRole>
         <id root='…' extension='SPM-2'/>
         <specimenPlayingEntity>
            <code code='SPM-4' … >
               <qualifier>
                  <name nullFlavor='NA'>
                     <originalText
                        >Modifier</originalText></name>
                  <value code='SPM-5'/>
               </qualifier>
               <qualifier>
                  <name nullFlavor='NA'>
                     <originalText
                        >Additive</originalText></name>
                  <value code='SPM-6'/>
               </qualifier>
            </code>
            <quantity value='SPM-12.1' unit='SPM-12.2'/>
            <name></name>
            <desc>SPM-14</desc>
         </specimenPlayingEntity>
      </specimenRole>
   </specimen>
</procedure>
```

Fig. 17.26 SPM mapping to CDA specimen and procedure

Specimen ID (SPM-2)

This field contains the identifier of the specimen and should be mapped to the <id> element of the <specimenRole>.

Specimen Type (SPM-4)

This field identifies the type of specimen. It should be placed in the `<code>` element of the `<specimenPlayingEntity>`.

Specimen Type Modifier (SPM-5)

This field may be used to identify a subtype for the specimen when SPM-4 is insufficient to fully identify the specimen type. This should be mapped to a `<name>` element of the `<qualifier>` in the `<code>` element under `<specimenPlayingEntity>`. The `<name>` element in the `<qualifier>` element indicates that this code is a modifier.

Specimen Additives (SPM-6)

This field may be used to identify additives to the specimen. This can be mapped to a `<name>` element of the `<qualifier>` in the `<code>` element under `<specimen-PlayingEntity>`. The `<name>` element in the `<qualifier>` element indicates that this code is for additives.

Specimen Collection Method (SPM-7)

This field identifies the method used to collect the specimen and appears in the `<code>` element of the `<procedure>` that describes how the specimen was collected.

Specimen Source Site (SPM-8) and Specimen Source Site Modifier (SPM-9)

SPM-8 and SPM-9 identify the site the specimen was taken from. The SPM-8 field is mapped to the code XML attribute the `<targetSiteCode>` element. SPM-9 may be used in the code XML attribute on the `<value>` element found in the `<qualifier>` of the `<code>`. The `<name>` element of this `<qualifier>` should indicate that this code is a modifier.

Specimen Collection Site (SPM-10)

The collection site indicates the site used to approach the target site and so is mapped to the code XML attribute of the `<approachSiteCode>` in the `<procedure>` element.

Specimen Collection Amount (SPM-12)

The quantity of specimen collected appears in this field. It should be mapped to the `<quantity>` element of the `<specimenPlayingEntity>`. The first component of this field should appear in the value XML attribute. The second component should be mapped to the unit XML attribute.

Specimen Description (SPM-14)

This field describes the specimen, and should appear in the `<desc>` element under the `<specimenPlayingEntity>` element.

Specimen Collection Date/Time (SPM-17)

This field is the time at which the specimen collection procedure was performed. It appears in the value XML attribute of the `<effectiveTime>` element in the `<procedure>`.

Fields Not Mapped

Details about specimen handling, its relationship to other specimens, the container, and an evaluation of the specimen with regard to condition or quality are not supported by the CDA standard. Details necessary to manage the transport or delivery of the specimen are also not provided. Most of these details are to support the workflow in the laboratory and are not relevant to the report on the result.

Summary

- The HL7 Version 2 ORU, MDM and ADT messages can be converted into CDA documents.
- One way to convert an HL7 Version 2 message is to translate it into its XML equivalent and then use XSLT to translate it into a CDA document.
- Most HL7 Version 2 data types have a straightforward mapping to an HL7 Version 3 data type.
- The OBX segment usually maps to a CDA `<observation>` unless used in an MDM message, in which case it might represent the `<text>` element in the `<nonXMLBody>`.
- The TXA segment fills in details of the `<ClinicalDocument>` element.
- The PID segment corresponds to the `<recordTarget>` element in CDA.
- The PV1 segment maps to the `<encompassingEncounter>` element in the CDA header.

- The NK1 segment maps to `<participant>` elements in the CDA header.
- The MSH and EVN segments can be used as a source of information regarding important times an identifiers needed in the CDA Header.
- The ORC segment supplies information that can appear in the `<infulfillmentOf>` or the `<encounterPartcipant>` elements in the CDA header.
- The OBR segment can map to a `<section>` or to an `<observation>` element, or both.
- The NTE segment represents a comment or annotation. This should use the CCD form for comments.
- The SPM segment represents a `<specimen>` participant in a clinical statement. It also contains information about the `<procedure>` used to collect the specimen.

Questions

1. What segment most closely resembles the CDA Header?
2. What segment is primarily mapped to elements beneath the `<patientRole>` element?
3. What CDA element would a PV1 segment be mapped to?
4. What segment requires the deepest understanding of the business rules for creating messages that use it?
5. What Version 2 message would contain the content for the `<nonXMLBody>` element?
6. How would you represent the role of a patient contact found in an NK1 segment in a CDA document?
7. What segment could influence both the `<section>` and the clinical statements appearing below it?
8. If the CDA document being produced uses other CCD templates, what clinical statement element should be used to represent the content of an NTE segment?

Research Questions

Chapter 8 on Observation Reporting of the HL7 Version 2 standard contains a number of sample narrative report messages.

1. Select an appropriate message from this chapter (or another source) and convert it to a CDA Level 1 document.
2. Select an appropriate message from this chapter (or another source) and convert it to a CDA Level 2 document.
3. Convert a laboratory report message in ORU format to a CDA Level 3 document.*

Extracting Data from a CDA™ Document 18

18.1
Data Extraction

At least two open source APIs exist to read CDA clinical documents into an object model in memory. The general pattern is to create a Clinical Document object in memory, initialize it from a CDA document, and then begin to access the components of the model using various setter and getter methods. The CDAPI from Mirth Corporation is one open source project that supports this. It makes use of the CDA Tools work developed in the Model Driven Health Tools Project of Open Health Tools.

A very similar way to do this uses the raw XML APIs that are common to most programming environments. In this case, an XML Document object is created in memory that conforms to the W3C DOM standard. This object is initialized from the CDA document. Components of the model are accessed directly using XPath statements, or through programmatic traversal of the XML document.

18.2
XPath Searching Through Context

One challenge in using XPath is that context propagates downwards through the CDA XML representation. This means that you need a moderately complex XPath 1.0 expression to retrieve the context components regardless of what level they are declared in the document. For example, the author of clinical statement might be defined in the `<ClinicalDocument>`, `<section>`, a clinical statement in the `<entry>`, or any clinical statement in an `<entryRelationship>` elements that appear "above" the clinical statement being examined in the document hierarchy, or in the clinical statement itself. To locate the author, you must first look to see if any authors are declared in the clinical statement being examined. If there are none there, you must look above at the next point, and so forth, until you reach the top of the document.

The following XPath 1.0 expression accomplishes this task quite handily, but it needs some explanation.

```
ancestor-or-self::*[cda:author][1]/cda:author
```

The ancestor-or-self:: pattern appearing in the XPath expression above means "Look in this element and in all of its ancestors for the pattern that follows", and return results in

K.W. Boone, *The CDA™ Book*,   261
DOI: 10.1007/978-0-85729-336-7_18, © Springer-Verlag London Limited 2011

reverse document order. The next part of the pattern * simply means look at every element. The next part of the pattern [cda:author] qualifies the previous part, essentially saying "but only if it contains at least one <author> element". The next part of the XPath expression says "take the first element of the set given by the previous expression". The last part cda:author asks for all <author> elements that are children of the element found.

Putting all that together, the expression is interpreted to mean "Find the first element from right here (the clinical statement being examined) to the top of the document that contains at least one author, and list all of the <author> elements it contains."

This expression works perfectly fine if the contextConductionInd XML attribute is never set to false in the <entryRelationship> or <component> element. When contextConductionInd is set to false, the examination loop has to stop after that element is examined.

To complete the search when the contextConductionInd XML attribute can be false requires either a two step search process, or the use of a more powerful searching language, such as XPath 2.0 or XQuery.

There are some advanced XSLT tricks that can be used to determine if the author element attempts to traverse the broken context, but these are left as a research exercise at the end of this chapter.

Summary

- Extracting data can be done through code using model based open source APIs.
- Data can also be extracted using the XML DOM and XPath Expressions.
- Data Extraction needs to search through context for some data elements.
- Setting contextConductionInd XML attribute to false in the <entryRelationship> can make some extraction tasks more complex.

Questions

1. Which association classes in CDA permit a change in how context is conducted?
2. What XPath expression could you use to extract the relevant <informant> elements associated with a clinical statement?

Research Questions

1. What open Source APIs can you find to read a CDA Document?
2. How would you use XSLT to detect that an <author> element in an ancestor of a clinical statement was not conducted down to a child element?*
3. How would you accomplish this using an API that supported CDA? Does the API support navigation through the context?*

Templates

19

According to §1.1 of the HL7 Templates DSTU:

> *A template is an expression of a set of constraints on the RIM or a RIM derived model that is used to apply additional constraints to a portion of an instance of data which is expressed in terms of some other Static Model. Templates are used to further define and refine these existing models to specify a narrower and more focused scope.*

Put more simply: A template is a collection of business rules which are applied to part of a document or message and which are defined to meet the needs of a specific use case.

Templates can be defined in a number of ways. They can be created using HL7 modeling tools, UML modeling tools, as human readable specifications, or in other machine-processable forms such as ISO Schematron.

By far the most common method of defining templates is to use human readable specifications, augmented by ISO Schematron for validation.

While the HL7 Template Draft Standard for Trial Use (DSTU) goes into much more detail, it has expired and is in the process of being updated. The following general principles are derived in part from that DSTU, and are based on the best practices established by the various organizations developing templates, including HL7 Structured Documents, Integrating the Healthcare Enterprise, and ANSI/HITSP.

Every template has a unique identifier. An instance that asserts conformance to a template in some class adds a `<templateId>` element to that class.

When the templates are constructed using HL7 modeling tools, the HL7 Model identifier appears in the extension attribute of the `<templateId>` element. The `root` attribute contains the value 2.16.840.1.113883.1.3 which is the OID for the namespace used for HL7 models. Templates not created using HL7 modeling tools are usually assigned an OID. This is considered to be the best practice according to the HL7 Structured Documents Workgroup, and has been followed subsequently by other organizations.

Each template represents a set of constraints on a model. However, it has been subsequently discovered that a set of templates designed for the CDA™ model (specifically those on entries in the HL7 Continuity of Care Document or CCD) could also be applied to other models, such as those found in the HL7 Care Record DSTU. Simply put, a set of constraints can be applied to any model that permits them to be applied, unless the template itself prohibits that use.

One of the reasons that CCD templates could be applied to the HL7 Care Record DSTU is that both of them have the clinical statement model in common. While there are a few minor variations between the models, nothing was done that prohibits the application of a

K.W. Boone, *The CDA™ Book*,
DOI: 10.1007/978-0-85729-336-7_19, © Springer-Verlag London Limited 2011

CCD template to the Care Record. There are for example, no requirements to include data in the CCD that cannot be included in the Care Record.

More than one template can be used at the same time in the same place. The only requirement is that all rules for each template are followed. Templates can be layered, so that one template depends on and requires the use of another for the same part. This is essentially the principal of inheritance. IHE can define a template that builds from an HL7 template and adds new rules without having to copy all of the rules from the HL7 template. It simply requires that an instance that conforms to a particular IHE template also conform to a less constrained HL7 template.

This provides another way to support incremental interoperability. Each layer provides a more constrained view of the data being exchanged. If a system supports template A and a more constrained template B, then when it communicates with a system that understands the more constrained version, a high level of interoperability is achieved. But if the other system only understands template A, then some interoperability is achieved, just not perhaps as much as could be obtained.

The use of inheritance in templates works best when an open model of exchange is being used. That model of exchange is one where the sender and receiver agree upon a set of data to exchange that will be processed in certain ways. They also agree that the sender can send more than the receiver might be able to process, and that it is acceptable for the receiver to ignore this information. An example of this would be in the exchange of problems, where sender and receiver agree to use a certain code set to identify problems, but where the sender also sends their local code. The receiver need not understand or process that information in order for the exchange to be successful.

This is a use of open templates. *Open templates permit anything to be done in the underlying standard that is not explicitly prohibited.* This allows templates to be built up over time that extend and go beyond the original use cases for which they were originally designed.

Closed templates only permit what has been defined in the template, and do not permit anything beyond that. There are good reasons to use closed templates, sometimes having to do with local policy. For example, in communicating information from a healthcare provider to a public health agency, some information may need to be omitted to ensure patient privacy laws are followed.

Most templates developed for CDA are of the open sort.

Another consideration with templates is how deep the template should go. A model is a collection of classes and associations between them, so a single template could produce constraints on several different classes. In actual practice, most templates that have been developed are rather shallow. The template itself describes what must be present in the class, and what associations are used. But it then simply requires that associated classes conform to another template.

This creates a somewhat recursive or "fractal" model of templates. The document is a template that requires the presence of several section templates. Each section template might require the presence of subsection templates, or entry templates, or both. An entry template might then require a clinical statement to be associated with another clinical statement that conforms to yet another template.

Being able to break a large model down into a variety of smaller, reusable set of constraints has proven to be very valuable, and is one that I strongly recommend.

19.1
Building Implementation Guides Using Templates

Building a CDA Implementation Guide is usually executed in a top down fashion. The first step is to identify the kind of document you are creating. Then you develop requirements for the document header, body and clinical statements, usually in that order. Templates are often created for at each level to keep requirements modular and easy to manage and to make the components reusable in other projects.

The Document Template

The first step in creating the document template is often determining what kind of clinical document is being generated. This creates requirements on what appears in `<code>` element used to generate the clinical document.

The next step determines which of the participants and act relationships in the header must or should be present. These requirements are determined based upon the use case. For example, a template for a clinical document describing the results of a laboratory report might require information about the clinical lab which produced the results in the header. This would result in a requirement that a `<serviceEvent>` element be present, and that `<serviceEvent>` be used to record the information about the performing lab in a `<performer>` element.

The final step for the document template is to determine what must appear in the body of the clinical document. In some cases, this requirement might just be for non-structured content, in which case the requirements might specify a particular MIME type, encoding, et cetera, of the content which might be used in the `<nonXMLBody>`.

In other cases, the requirement would be for structured narrative to appear in the `<structuredBody>` element. Requirements may be derived from specific needs identified in the use case. They also may be set, as has been done for some guides, by analyzing what occurs in current practice, and using that as a baseline to set requirements. The end result of this step is a list of sections that may, should or shall be included in the clinical document. The set of sections that appear in the clinical document are specified as business rules associated with the clinical document, and are then attached to the template for that document.

Header Templates

Each participant or act that helps to set the context of the clinical document in the CDA header can also be further constrained. Usually these constraints are set upon the association classes (participations and act relationships). They usually include constraints on the included role or act classes. Using the lab example above, the use case requires that the organization performing the test, and a person responsible for oversight of tests performed at that organization be sent in documents communicating laboratory results. It further requires that the organization identifier be present using a nationally specified identifier, and that contact information (address and phone number) be included in the communication.

Thus, two new templates are developed. One is produced for the `<performer>` elements describing the organization that ran the tests, and the supervising person, and requires that the organization ID be sent a certain way, and that the address and telephone be sent using non-empty values. Another template is created that ensures that the service event itself contains the required performer template, and includes required details about the service performed and the dates of service.

Section Templates

The content of each section is then evaluated. If the section just contains narrative, the business rules should at least indicate what kind of information should be present in the narrative. In other cases, there may be requirements that the section include certain entries. These are attached as business rules to the section.

Requirements on the section typically include the code used to identify the section, and required or optional subsections or entries. On occasion there may be a need to specify business rules on the various participations in the section. For example, in developing an implementation guide for a labor and delivery summary, IHE determined that the section in the delivery record describing the baby must have a `<subject>` participation that identified the baby and provided the baby's demographic information.

Entry Templates

Today, most of the entry templates that a use case would need have already been developed. There are a few cases where they have not, and these are most often dealing with collections of structured results. In these cases, most often the effort involves determining what information needs to be gathered together and organizing it in some way.

Should you encounter a case where you need a use case specific entry template, these are the steps that you would normally follow.

1. Determine the type of clinical statement needed. Is this template for a procedure, encounter, observation, act, et cetera?
2. Identify the code system and code value or value set that will be used to identify this particular act or clinical statement. This will place requirements on `<code>`.
3. Determine the key piece of information to be returned. Then identify the appropriate data type to represent that information. Look at all the places where that data type presently appears in the CDA Clinical Statement model. More often than not, that will help to identify where the data will go.
4. Determine what details will be recorded. There are some very simple questions to ask, and each of these questions will place requirements on the different parts of the clinical statement.

Who	Questions of who is involved or affected by a clinical statement place requirements upon the participants in the clinical statement.
What	Questions of what need to be looked at further. If the answer to what is a description of an action to be performed, then it usually places requirements on the `<code>` element of the clinical statement. On the other hand, if the answer is a noun, then it may be a participant (e.g., a medication, a specimen, et cetera).
Where	Questions of where describe locations, and these are participants where the type of participant is a location. See Encounter Location on page 145 for an example.
When	Questions of when will involve the time data type, and will usually appear either in the `<time>` element of the participation or the `<effectiveTime>` for the clinical statement. Be wary of including time as a `<value>` in an `<observation>` element.
Why	Questions of why are associated with reasoning or causation linking two clinical statements. The `<entryRelationship>` element is the most common way to link two clinical statements. The possible answers to these questions place requirements for relationships between acts to be recorded in an `<entryRelationship>` element. They also often require the `classCode` XML attribute of the `<entryRelationship>` to be RSON, CAUS or MFST representing reasons, causes or manifestations respectively.
How	Answers to these questions usually reflect on the method that something is done. This again would be related to describing the act being performed, and would be associated with the type of clinical statement and its `<code>` element.

Building upon Other Implementation Guides

There have been over 500 templates developed in existing CDA implementation guides. HL7, IHE, ANSI/HITSP, epSOS, and Continua have defined about 50 document templates, more than 100 section templates, and another 100 entry templates. Numerous other organizations have defined their own CDA templates. In almost all cases these organizations have reused templates from other specifications (Of course you have to start somewhere. The HL7 Continuity of Care Document is the most often referenced guide and it defined most of the templates that are refined or reused elsewhere.).

Because there are so many templates, it can be difficult to find them. HL7 is working upon a template registry that will eventually make this easier. Until then, the best thing to do is send a question to the HL7 Structured Documents workgroup e-mail list. The table below shows where you can go to find a number of different implementation guides for CDA templates. This is not a complete list, but is a good place to start.

Table 19.1 Template sources

Organization	Website
Health Level 7	http://www.hl7.org
Integrating the Healthcare Enterprise	http://www.ihe.net
epSOS	http://www.epsos.eu/
Health Story	http://healthstory.com
ANSI/HITSP	http://www.hitsp.org

Some of these templates are described briefly in Chap. 21 below. More often than not, most use cases can use templates that have already been defined for entries.

Types of Constraints

Most constraints on CDA implementation guides apply to the sender or creator of a clinical document rather than how the receiver of the clinical document uses that information. There are cases where the CDA document is used as part of a clinical workflow, and so implementation guide developers should consider these issues as well. The language around constraints can sometimes be confusing and open to interpretation. Template specifications should be very clear on how they define terms used for requirements. The IETF RFC-2119 is a good example of how to define terms, and is used by many standards development organizations. This specification can be found on the web at http://www.ietf.org/rfc/rfc2119.txt. To use these definitions in your implementation guide you need only insert the following phrase near the beginning of your guide:

> The key words "MUST", "MUST NOT", "REQUIRED", "SHALL", "SHALL NOT", "SHOULD", "SHOULD NOT", "RECOMMENDED", "MAY", and "OPTIONAL" in this document are to be interpreted as described in RFC 2119.

It is also important to visibly distinguish requirements of an implementation guide from other explanatory text so that implementers can find requirements. Key words such as those above are often highlighted when used in conformance constraints.

Mandatory

Mandatory constraints require both the data element and its content to be included in the document. These are most often stated using terms such as SHALL, MUST, or REQUIRED on both the data element and its content. The data can never be sent using a flavor of null.

Required

These constraints require the data element to be sent, but allow its content to be a flavor of null in exceptional cases (e.g., an unidentified patient, where demographics are unknown). These are most often stated using SHALL, MUST, or REQUIRED on the data element. The content may be a flavor of null in exceptional cases

Conditional

Conditional constraints require an application to send data when certain conditions are met. These are typically stated using SHALL, MUST or REQUIRED on the data element or its content under certain conditions which must be specified.

Required If Known

These are often stated as SHOULD or RECOMMENDED. However, the preferred way to state these is as a conditional requirement where the condition is "when known". The sender must be able to demonstrate the capability to send this information, but there may be cases where the information is not present, applicable or known and so the document may not always contain it.

Recommended

Constraints of this form recommend behavior based on recognized best practices. These are often used when some systems are unable to conform to best practices because of other limitations.

These constraints are often indicated using terms such as SHOULD or RECOMMENDED.

Optional

Constraints of this form indicate expected behavior should the sender choose to send certain information. An optional constraint should be viewed as a requirement to do something a certain way when it is done, but not require that it be done. For example, it may be optional to send coded vital signs using a certain template according to an implementation guide. This should be viewed as it is optional to send the vital signs in a coded form, but a requirement that when coded vital signs are sent, that they do conform to the specified template. These requirements are often indicated using terms such as OPTIONAL, PERMITTED or MAY. In some cases, the constraint is stated in the negative. In these cases, the phrase NEED NOT is preferred over MAY NOT, because the latter is ambiguously interpreted as an option or a prohibition.

Not Recommended

Some systems may behave in ways that are not considered to be best practice, but have no other choice. To allow for the behavior of these systems, constraints are often written in this form to indicate an acceptable behavior that is known to be other than the best practice. Constraints of this form are often written using terms such as NOT RECOMMENDED, or SHOULD NOT.

Prohibited

Constraints of this form are absolute prohibitions. For example, in some countries, information on religion, race, and ethnicity cannot be transmitted by law. This would result in a constraint that prohibits the use of certain data elements in a transmission.

Table 19.2 Requirements on vital signs

Code	Display name	UCUM unit	Datatype
9279-1	RESPIRATION RATE	/min	PQ
8867-4	HEART BEAT	/min	PQ
2710-2	OXYGEN SATURATION	%	PQ
8480-6	INTRAVASCULAR SYSTOLIC	mm[Hg]	PQ
8462-4	INTRAVASCULAR DIASTOLIC	mm[Hg]	PQ
8310-5	BODY TEMPERATURE	Cel or [degF]	PQ
8302-2	BODY HEIGHT (MEASURED)	m, cm, [in_us] or [in_uk]	PQ
3141-9	BODY WEIGHT (MEASURED)	kg, g, [lb_av] or [oz_av]	PQ

This table is derived from content appearing in the IHE PCC Technical Framework Volume 2, Revision 6.0.

These constraints are often written using terms such as SHALL NOT, NOT PERMITTED, or MUST NOT. The phrase NOT REQUIRED is not used as it implies optional.

Co-occurrence

Constraints on information are usually one a single data item. Co-occurrence constraints deal with relationships between two or more data items. These sometimes appear in a tabular form, where requirements in each column address different data elements that are sent. For example, Table 19.2 above shows an example where vital signs are required to be reported a certain way.

These can also be written in a conditional form, as in: "If the data item being sent is the patient's weight, it shall be sent in kilograms", or "When the observation is a diagnosis, it shall be sent using a diagnosis code from ICD-10".

19.2
CDA Extensions

At times you will find that the CDA standard does not immediately support something that your use case requires you to record. Fortunately the CDA standard allows for extension to meet this sort of requirement. According to the standard, you are permitted to include elements from a namespace other than urn:hl7-org:v3 in the CDA document. In Section [§1.4] the standard states "*Locally-defined markup may be used when local semantics have no corresponding representation in the CDA specification.*"

Be aware that many implementations may (incorrectly according to the standard) fail to recognize a document containing an extension element as a valid CDA document. The next chapter describes how implementations can validate a CDA document even when extension elements are present.

Over time, HL7 and other organizations have come to establish best practices to be used in the development of extensions to the CDA standard. The principals established make use of the HL7 Reference Implementation Model.

1. Extensions should be optional rather than required or mandatory. This may not be possible for all use cases.
2. Extensions defined in a single implementation guide should appear in a common namespace.
3. The namespace in which an extension appears must be defined.
4. The extension element should use existing HL7 data types and vocabularies where possible. Note that the ED data type allows for arbitrary MIME content, which means that there is relatively little content that would not be allowed under this requirement.
5. The extension should be drawn from the HL7 RIM where feasible, and use the RIM data element name.
6. Many guides require that the extension element appear in the location where it would appear had the data element been part of the CDA standard.

To see how these requirements would be applied, let us take the requirement that a CDA document be digitally signed by the legal authenticator.

In the HL7 RIM, there is a class attribute on the `participation` class called `signatureText`. This class attribute is defined as being "A textual or multimedia depiction of the signature by which the participant endorses his or her participation in the Act …" [§RIM 3.1.3.11].

A digital signature can be represented in an XML document using the XML Signature and Syntax standard from the W3C. To represent this content in a CDA document, you would need to allow for a `<ext:signatureText>` element to appear after the `<cda:signatureCode>` element, and to further specify how the contents of this extension element would be formatted.

Use of this extension element could require senders and receivers to modify the XML schemas they use to validate their CDA document, which is one reason why the rules above recommend that extension elements be optional.

There are cases where extension under the rules above would seem to be prohibited. These cases involve restriction on vocabulary used with existing act relationships, participations, et cetera. For example, the current version of the HL7 Version 3 RIM includes a mood code of RSK that can be used to identify acts that might occur in the future but which are undesirable. A Risk can be viewed as being the opposite of a goal. An application desiring to record patient risks using `<cda:observation>` elements that include this value in the XML moodCode attribute could not do so directly following the recommendations above.

There are two ways to address this using the extension mechanism. The first of these is to define an `<ext:observation>` element that is defined in the same way that the `<cda:observation>` is defined with the exception that the moodCode attribute is permitted to contain the value RSK. The second way only works when the requirement is to use a new vocabulary term that is a refinement of an existing term allowed by the standard.

For example, the HL7 Patient Care workgroup defined a new subtype of observation (OBS) known as a Concern (CONC). A use case may require that concerns represented in an `<observation>` be specifically identified. This could be accomplished by defining an extension attribute `ext:classCode` that could appear on `<cda:observation>`. That extension would provide more detail about the subtype of observation. Again, this only works when the new vocabulary term is a subtype of an existing term, because the existing term would still be used in the transmission. A use of this form is shown in the figure below.

```
<cda:observation classCode='OBS' ext:classCode='CONC'/>
```

Where Should Extensions Go?

The last recommendation in the list above has been defined as a best practice by many organizations (including the HL7 Structured Docuements workgroup). However, it may not be ideal. Requiring an extension element to appear where it "should have" appeared in the standard makes it nearly impossible to create a CDA schema that can validate a legal CDA document containing a legal extension. There are too many places where these elements could appear, and modifying the schemas would produce a messy, and possibly even invalid schema, because it could be non-deterministic.

It would be relatively easy to extend the CDA schema to allow extension elements by appending a two schema declarations at the end of each element declaration. The first would allow any extension element, and the second any extension attribute. These schema declarations would allow elements from a foreign namespace to appear at the end of the element.

Figure 19.1 shows a slightly modified schema definition for the CDA <observationRange> element. This illustrates the mechanism for adding extension

```
<xs:complexType name="POCD_MT000040.ObservationRange">
  <xs:sequence>
      <xs:element name="realmCode" type="CS"
          minOccurs="0" maxOccurs="unbounded"/>
      <xs:element name="typeId" minOccurs="0"
          type="POCD_MT000040.InfrastructureRoot.typeId" />
      <xs:element name="templateId" type="II"
          minOccurs="0" maxOccurs="unbounded"/>
      <xs:element name="code" type="CD" minOccurs="0"/>
      <xs:element name="text" type="ED" minOccurs="0"/>
      <xs:element name="value" type="ANY" minOccurs="0"/>
      <xs:element name="interpretationCode" type="CE"
          minOccurs="0"/>
      <xs:any namespace="##other" processContents="skip"
          minOccurs="0" maxOccurs="unbounded"
      />
  </xs:sequence>
  <xs:attribute name="nullFlavor"
      type="NullFlavor" use="optional"/>
  <xs:attribute name="classCode"
      type="ActClassObservation"
      use="optional" default="OBS"/>
  <xs:attribute name="moodCode" type="ActMood"
      use="optional" fixed="EVN.CRT"/>
  <xs:anyAttribute namespace="##other"/>
</xs:complexType>
```

Fig. 19.1 Adding extension support to a CDA schema

support to the existing schemas. This schema declaration allows extension elements and attributes to appear within the contents of a CDA document in a way that allows it to be validated using the standard schema.

Summary

- A template is a set of uniquely identified business rules that apply to part of a CDA document to meet a specific need.
- The templates that are applied to an element in a CDA document are identified in the `<templateId>` element.
- Templates can be defined in a number of ways. By far the most common is through a text specification.
- More than one template can be applied to part of a CDA document at the same time so long as the rules do not conflict with each other.
- Templates can inherit rules from other templates easily and without duplicating the rules by simply requiring that the other template to be used.
- A template can be applied to a variety of different messages so long as they support the same semantic models.
- Reuse of templates can save quite of bit of time in developing specifications.
- Most templates address a single class or an association class and its nearest members.
- Constructing a template usually, but not always, follows a top down refinement process.
- When building a template, consider what requirements address, who, what, where, when, why and how.
- There are numerous implementation guides and templates already developed for CDA.
- Extensions to CDA are permitted, and may be necessary when a use case has requirements that cannot be modeled using the standard.
- Putting extensions at the end of an item defined by the CDA standard makes it easier to validate the CDA document according to an XML schema.

Questions

1. What XML element identifies the business rules that a component of a CDA document follows?
2. "The clinical document header MUST contain an `<assignedAuthoringDevice>` element to represent the device that produced the ECG, and the information on that device must be present" is an example of what kind of constraint?
3. True or false: HL7 requires use of a specific language to specify a template.
4. True or false: A template cannot be applied to anything other than the HL7 artifact it was written for.
5. True or false: If the template does not define how to do something, it is not permitted.

Research Questions

1. Where would you look to find existing templates. How many document templates did you find? Sections? Entries?
2. Find a sample document produced by an EHR system (At least one is good, several would be better. Ensure that the documents you are using do not contain information from real patients.). Produce an implementation guide from this example using templates.*

Validating the Content of a CDA™ Document

20

Validation is the process of ensuring that something conforms to the requirements for it. In the context of XML, an XML document is valid if it conforms to the schema defined for it. The most commonly used schema these days is the W3C XML Schema standard. The CDA standard provides a schema using the W3C XML Schema standard that can be used for validation.

According to the CDA standard, an instance is not valid if it does not conform to the CDA schema.

There are however, several requirements defined in the CDA standard that either cannot be validated using an XML Schema, or which have not been incorporated into the schema delivered with the CDA standard. In many cases, an XML element must have one attribute or another but not both. This sort of constraint cannot even be represented in XML Schema, but can be represented in other schema languages.

There are other invalid cases that are not detected by the CDA schema. Many of these could have been addressed, but would have required hand editing of the machine generated schemas that the HL7 tools created automatically for CDA. In most of these cases, the value of maintaining these modifications was deemed to be less valuable than being able to support ongoing development efforts.

For example, the `<value>` elements in a `<regionOfInterest>` element must always be paired because they represent points on a plane. This could have been addressed in the CDA schema but was not because it would have required hand editing the schema. Similarly, the `<text>` element of the `<parentDocument>` can never contain text by value, it must always use the `<reference>` element to point to the location where the parent document can be found.

The constraints just described can be validated using a number of different XML based tools. ISO Schematron is a standard XML language based on XPath and XSLT that supports detection of certain kinds of patterns in XML documents. It can be, and has been used extensively, to detect violations of business rules. It is also used inside HL7 Version 3 XML schemas for data types to detect violations that are not easily detected using the W3C Schema standard.

Model based validation tools work by representing the CDA model in the RIM, using either the HL7 Model Interchange Format, or in UML. In some cases, these tools allow additional constraints to be associated with templates. The Model Driven Health Tools project in the Open Health Tools open source initiative is one example of a model based validation tool.

Validation is made more difficult by the XML ITS approach to extensions on the RIM. Content in the XML document that is not in the urn:hl7-org:v3 namespace is assumed to be a local extension to the standard. There are very few additional rules about where these

K.W. Boone, *The CDA™ Book*,
DOI: 10.1007/978-0-85729-336-7_20, © Springer-Verlag London Limited 2011

extensions can appear, which makes it impossible to craft a W3C XML Schema for any HL7 Version 3 standard (including CDA), that allows extensions wherever they may be present. Other techniques must be used to validate the CDA content when extensions are present. The content in the extension may also need to be validated.

20.1
Using the CDA Schemas

Validating a CDA document using the W3C XML Schemas is very easy. Most XML pars-ers include the capability to validate using an XML Schema. You must first obtain a copy of the CDA schemas. These are part of the CDA standard, which can be obtained from HL7 International. You must tell the parser where the schema is located on your system, read it in and enable the validation capability.

When using a validating parser, there are a couple of items that you should check for in the CDA document first. If the CDA document contains the XML Schema `xsi:schemaLocation` attribute on the root element, this should be removed. Technically, this would not be a valid CDA document because the XML ITS prohibits use of this attribute. However, it is a fairly common error that still appears in many implementations. If you received the CDA document from a foreign source, this loca-tion very likely does not exist on your system. Even if the location were a publically accessible URL, you should still remove it. Your application should only use CDA schemas that it controls, not a schema under the control of an outside source.

After configuring the parser, and ensuring that the CDA document instance does not contain an `xsi:schemaLocation` attribute, you can then parse the document.

There are other advantages of using a validating parser. Parsing the CDA document in this fashion will ensure that all fixed and default values are automatically inserted by the parser if they were not present in the CDA document instance.

20.2
ISO Schematron

ISO Schematron can be used in two different ways to assist in validating a CDA docu-ment. Schematron rules can be added to the W3C Schema if your validating parser sup-ports this technique. Schematron.NET is one implementation that supports this in the .NET environment.

One of the benefits of the ISO Schematron standard is that it can be implemented using an XSLT transformation. That is not the only way to implement it, just the most common one. The base transformation is run over the Schematron schema. It produces an XSLT stylesheet that can then be used to process an input document to see if it follows the rules expressed in the Schematron schema.

The same technique can also be used to generate a set of Schematron rules using a W3C Sch-ema that contains embedded Schematron rules in `<appinfo>` elements of the W3C Schema.

Just about every modern development platform supports XSLT. This makes it very easy to use a Schematron schema to validate content. This is presently one of the most popular ways to validate conformance to CDA templates. There are over 30 CDA implementation guides that use Schematron for validation.

The National Institute for Standards and Technology (NIST) in the US has developed ISO Schematron rules for CDA implementation guides created by Integrating the Healthcare Enterprise and the ANSI Health Information Technology Standards Panel (HITSP). NIST also worked in conjunction with IHE, HITSP, Lantana Consulting Group, and the Certification Commission on Health IT (CCHIT) to create an online validation tool that supports many CDA implementation guides.

The NIST CDA Validator is available on the web at http://xreg2.nist.gov/cda-validation/index.html. Andrew McCaffrey of NIST was awarded the very first "Ad Hoc Harley" for his efforts in developing this tool, and working with all of the different organizations to ensure that it did the right thing.

Schematron rules are written as a collection assertions against a particular context within a CDA document. The context defines the location where the rule is executed, and is expressed in XPath notation. Assertions are also written as XPath expressions that must be true if the rule is to pass.

The example Schematron rule below can be used to validate conformance to the IHE History of Past Illness template.

```
<pattern name='Template_1.3.6.1.4.1.19376.1.5.3.1.3.6'>
 <rule context='*[cda:templateId/@root =
                "1.3.6.1.4.1.19376.1.5.3.1.3.6"]'>
   <!-- Verify the template is on the right object -->
   <assert test='../cda:section'>
     Error: This template can only be used on sections.
   </assert>
   <!-- Verify that required templates present. -->
   <assert test='cda:templateId[@root =
                "2.16.840.1.113883.10.20.1.11"]'>
     Error: The CCD template identifier for Problems
            is not present.
   </assert>
   <!-- Verify the section type code -->
   <assert test='cda:code[@code = "11450-4"]'>
     Error: The section type code must be 11450-4
   </assert>
   <assert test='cda:code[@codeSystem =
                "2.16.840.1.113883.6.1"]'>
     Error: The section type code must come from LOINC.
   </assert>
   <!-- Verify required data elements are present -->
   <assert test='.//cda:templateId[@root =
                "1.3.6.1.4.1.19376.1.5.3.1.4.5.2"]'>
     Error: The Active Problems Section must
            contain a Problem Concern Entry.
   </assert>
 </rule>
</pattern>
```

Fig. 20.1 A sample Schematron rule

The <rule> element sets the context of execution for the rule. In this case, the XPath expression indicates that the context is any element that asserts that it conforms to the template identified by 1.3.6.1.4.1.19376.1.5.3.1.3.8. In XML, this would be any element in the CDA document that contained the following in a child element.

```
<templateId root='1.3.6.1.4.1.19376.1.5.3.1.3.8'/>
```

Inside the <rule> element are several assertions. Each <assertion> element contains an XPath expression that must evaluate to true if the test is to pass. That XPath expression is evaluated in the context of the rule. If the XPath expression does not evaluate to true, then the Schematron processor emits the message contained inside the <assertion> element.

The rule above exhibits a number of features common to CDA Template implementations. The context of the rule is any element asserting that it conforms to a template. The rule is written this way to locate elements that may use a template incorrectly. If the search pattern had only looked for <section> elements containing the specified template, the test would not have discovered any other element that used it incorrectly. The first test ensures that the template is used on the correct element in the CDA instance.

The next rule ensures that any other required templates are present on the element. The next two rules ensure that a correct code and code system is used on a data element. The last rule ensures than any required templates are present in the child elements.

This rule demonstrates why multiple templates are often used in implementations. If template A defines a set of business rules, and template B is defined as being the set of rules in template A plus one more rule, implementation of template B can be done in two ways. Template B can copy every rule from template A and add a new rule. This can be rather challenging. Template B could also indicate that template A must be used along with the new rule. This latter case is demonstrated in the second of the tests shown in the rule above. The IHE template for the Active Problems section simply reuses the HL7 CCD template for the Problems section and adds a couple of additional rules. In fact, the tests on cda:code are completely unnecessary because the CCD template already has those rules. They are included here for illustration.

20.3
Model Based Validation

Model based validation is a technique whereby a computable model is stored. The CDA instance is validated against the constraints expressed in the computable model. If you think of XML Schema and ISO Schematron languages as computable representations of a model, you can see that this is simply a generalization of the schema validation techniques.

There are two common modeling forms in which model based validation is used. The HL7 Model Interchange Format (MIF) is a set of XML formats defined by the HL7 Tooling workgroup to support development of HL7 specifications, and is not really meant for human consumption. MIF is currently at Version 2.0 and is also being balloted by HL7 as a standard.

One MIF-based modeling tool used to validate CDA instances is the Eclipse CDA Editor. This editor runs in the Eclipse framework and can be used to edit and validate CDA instances. This is very useful for testing and development purposes but does not scale for validating instances in a production environment. The Eclipse CDA Editor is related to the H3ET project in the Eclipse Open Health Framework (OHF) open source project.

Off-the-shelf modeling tools more commonly based on UML and the OMG XML Metadata Interchange (XMI) standard often used to exchange UML models. Open Health Tools (OHT) has developed a project on Model Driven Health Tools. OHT seems to be at least the intellectual successor to the Eclipse OHF work, if not in fact the actual successor organization. This project has created models for many of the implementation guides described in Chap. 21. The project can be found on the web at http://cdatools.org. Dave Carleson of the VA was the fourth recipient of an "Ad Hoc Harley" for his efforts on the MDHT project.

The CDA tools project not only supports validation, but also creation of new templates, and the construction of Java code that can help read or create CDA documents.

20.4
Validating When CDA Extensions Are Used

Validating CDA in the presence of extensions can cause some difficulty because extensions do not appear in the Schema delivered with the CDA standard. It is also nearly impossible to create a CDA schema that supports every kind of extension allowed by the standard. You can often alter the CDA schema to support a fixed set of known extensions.

In order to validate a CDA document that can contain arbitrary extensions, you must do so in stages. The first stage should validate the extension content. This can be done using W3C Schema or ISO Schematron, or even code based validation. Having validated that the extension content is correctly formatted, it must now be removed from the CDA document before other validations can occur.

This can easily be done using a very small XSLT stylesheet. The stylesheet below copies all CDA elements, all attributes, and all text content, but does not copy any element from a foreign (non CDA) namespace.

```
<xsl:stylesheet
  xmlns:xsl='http://www.w3.org/1999/XSL/Transform'
  xmlns:cda='urn:hl7-org:v3'
  version='1.0'
>
  <xsl:template match="cda:*|text()|@*">
    <xsl:copy>
      <xsl:apply-templates select="cda:*|text()|@*"/>
    </xsl:copy>
  </xsl:template>
</xsl:stylesheet>
```

Fig. 20.2 Copying only CDA defined elements

This template can fail if your CDA document includes extension attributes, but this is rare. The simple solution is to include a new template that matches just the extension attribute and does nothing. If the extension attribute was `ext:myAttribute`, you would add the following line to the stylesheet.

```
<template match='ext:myAttribute'/>
```

20.5
Validating Narrative

Many implementation guides require that the content of a specific section be on the appropriate topic, e.g., that the History of Present Illness section contain a narrative summary of the events leading the current encounter. To verify that a system is capable of delivering appropriate content, you can test that it can send a message containing predefined strings of text. While this technique can be used to ensure that systems can deliver the required content, it cannot be used to ensure that the required kind of content is delivered in a production environment.

Summary

- CDA documents can be validated in a number of different ways.
- XML Schema cannot be used to validate all of the requirements of the CDA standard.
- Validating a CDA document that contains extensions can be done by first validating the extensions, removing them, and then validating the CDA document.
- You can verify that an implementation can produce appropriate narrative, but probably not in a production environment.

Questions

1. True or False: A CDA document that is valid according to the CDA XML schema is legal according to the CDA standard.
2. True or False: You can find the appropriate CDA schema to use for a document by inspecting the `xsi:schemaLocation` attribute.
3. Besides validating the content of a CDA document, what else will a validating parser do for your application?
4. True or false: ISO Schematron requires the use of XSLT.
5. True or false: You can use more than one schema language to validate a CDA document.
6. True or false: Model based validation is completely different from schema based validation.
7. True or false: MIF 2.0 is a standard format.
8. True or false: You cannot verify that a system can produce appropriate narrative content.
9. True or false: If an implementation requires the use of a particular extension, you will not be able to validate the CDA instances it sends using an XML Schema.

Research Questions

1. Where can you find the MIF representation for CDA Release 2.0?
2. Where can you find a UML representation of CDA Release 2.0?

Implementation Guides on CDA™   21

There are numerous implementation guides on CDA that have been developed around the world. The first CDA Release 2.0 implementation guide was published by in 2004 even before CDA Release 2.0 became an HL7 standard in 2005. Approximately 10% of the HL7 ballots over the last five years have been for CDA implementation guides. Since CDA Release 2.0 was published, over 100 implementation guides have been published using the standard.

The chart below shows the growth in both number of different CDA implementation guides and document types for which these specifications have been developed. A publication which describes two different document types counts as two guides in the chart below. This data includes CDA implementations for which guides have been published by HL7, IHE and ANSI/HITSP. There are numerous other guides which have been published by other organizations around the world which are not reflected in the chart below.

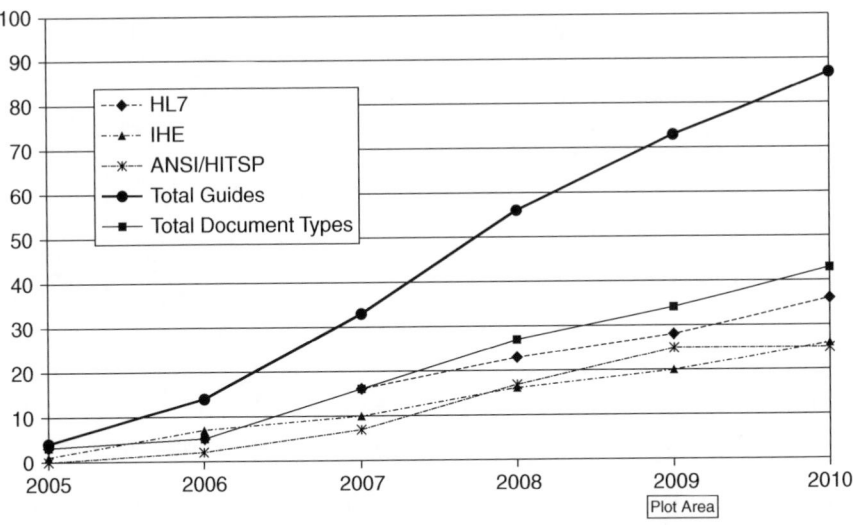

Fig. 21.1 CDA implementation guide growth

K.W. Boone, *The CDA™ Book*,   283
DOI: 10.1007/978-0-85729-336-7_21, © Springer-Verlag London Limited 2011

The sections below describe a number of different CDA implementation guides and provide some of the history behind them.

21.1
Claims Attachments (HL7)

The Claims Attachments Implementation Guides were started by HL7 in 1999 and were based on the CDA Release 1.0. These guides were intended to be used to meet requirements under US law to send clinical information in documents as attachments in insurance claims transactions. After almost 10 years, CMS finally produced a proposed regulation to meet the requirements that they do so, about 7 years after the deadline set by the Health Information Portability and Accountability Act (HIPAA). The regulation was never made final, and the current US PPACA Act now requires that such regulation be developed by 2014 (more than 15 years after the first act was passed requiring it).

Even though the use of Claims Attachment implementation guides never became a requirement under US regulation, they have greatly influenced the development of every CDA implementation guide produced subsequently. HL7 and Regenstrief Institute (the home of LOINC®) worked together to produce a document ontology that would live in the LOINC® terminology. The HL7 Document Ontology task force produced a collection of documents, and principals for their classification which produced an initial list of more than 50 document types. This list was loosely based on the encounter and management services that could be provided and billed for according to the CPT-4 Encounter and Management codes.

LOINC® and the Claims Attachment Workgroup in HL7 also produced a rather large list of components which could appear as sections within a clinical document. Almost every CDA Implementation Guide produced today is a beneficiary of that work.

From to early 2007 to early 2008, HL7 updated the Claims Attachment guides from CDA Release 1.0 to CDA Release 2.0. The first six publications from HL7 included more than 35 different document types (and are not reflected in the chart above). The HL7 Claims Attachment guides are some of the first guides to be produced, and so contain many original ideas. However, these guides adopted many of the lessons learned from later guides when they were revised in 2007.

21.2
Electronic Medical Summary (British Columbia/Vancouver Island Health Authority)

The first published implementation guide for CDA Release 2.0 is the Electronic Medical Summary (eMS) from British Columbia. This guide was produced to provide a specification for electronic medical summaries, and was published in final form in December of 2004. The intent was to create a specification that would be used by Electronic Medical Record systems to exchange medical summaries between physicians. The first published draft of this specification appeared in August of 2004 prior to the second to last ballot for CDA Release 2.0, and the final version was published before CDA Release 2.0 had even completed its final ballot cycle.

One of the most interesting aspects of this guide was its use of Schematron as a method to validate that a CDA document instance conformed to the specification. The demonstrated ability to automatically validate conformance to an implementation guide that this document showed was the reason that ISO Schematron has the preeminence it does today.

This guide described most of the requirements for the CDA in a tabular format similar to the HL7 Version 3 Hierarchical Description. It is also one of the few guides with any specific requirements on how the CDA narrative should appear.

The guide included sections for Problem List, Current Medications, Medical History, Surgical History, Family and Social History, Past Hospitalizations, Immunizations, Lab and Imaging Results, Imaging, and Height, Weight and Pulse.

21.3
Care Record Summary (HL7)

The idea for the HL7 Care Record Summary was first introduced to me in March of 2005. It was based on the work that had originally been developed for the e-MS guide described above. This guide was to support CDA Level 1 and Level 2. The document was created based on the LOINC sections used for the History and Physical Claims Attachment, and much of the work was done with a copy of the e-MS sitting beside my workstation while I edited the document. The eMS guide was shared with the HL7 Structured Documents Committee and we were encouraged to make use of it in this way. The first edition of the CRS was produced in less than 30 days, and that was mostly as a result of the preexisting claims attachment work, and the examples provided in the e-MS guide which were freely shared with HL7 Structured Documents by the publisher of that guide.

This guide was the subject of a great deal of disruption between the already difficult relations between HL7 and the ASTM E31 Health Informatics workgroup. ASTM threatened to sue HL7 for use of the materials they had developed for the ASTM Continuity of Care Record. They had believed that it would not have been possible to ballot a guide so quickly without having copied the work of the ASTM CCR. After several months, the threatened lawsuit was dropped. HL7 and ASTM agreed to resume active work jointly developing a new specification to be known as the Continuity of Care Document, based on the ASTM CCR and the HL7 CDA specification.

The CRS specification developed general principles for the CDA Header that were borrowed from the French Dossier Médical Personnel (DMP) project, and which were also present to some degree in the eMS specification from British Columbia. These principles required that the contact information for both the patient and other healthcare providers, including telephone numbers and addresses would appear in the CDA header.

The CRS included LOINC coded sections for Conditions (Problems), Allergies and Adverse Reactions, Medications, Hospital Course, Reason for Visit, Reason for Referral,

Advance Directives, History of Present Illness, Functional Status, Family and Social History, Immunizations, Surgical History, Prior Encounters, Review of Systems, Physical Examinations, Past Studies, and the Care Plan.

After work began on the Continuity of Care Document, HL7 and IHE began using it, and slowly the use of the Care Record Summary was discontinued. HL7 published a new version of the CRS as a DSTU in December of 2009, developed by the Health Story project, to ensure that there would be an implementation guide for Discharge Summaries, something that the Continuity of Care Document does not support. That work was informed by the original CRS specification, the Continuity of Care Document, and implementation guides developed by ANSI/HITSP.

21.4
Volet Médical (DMP)

The Volet Médical was a project of Le Dossier Médical Personnel (DMP). This work included a guide on the creation of the CDA Header, and the guide on the Medical Summary known as the Volet Médical. These documents were started in May of 2005. The Volet Médical required the use of the implementation guide for the header.

The implementation guide for the CDA Header required that all persons (patients and healthcare professionals) be identified in the CDA document header, and included the requirements that the person's name, identifier, address, and telephone number be included in the document.

These requirements were also included in the HL7 Care Record Summary implementation guide.

The Volet Médical included CDA sections for Health History, History of Past Illnesses, Surgical History, Psychiatric History, Pregnancy Status, General History, Family History, Allergies, Problems, Current Medications, Procedures, and Physical Examination Findings.

Implementation guides from the DMP project, as well as guides from many other international projects can be found on the excellent HL7 Book website maintained by René Spronk. That website can be found at http://hl7book.net/index.php?title=CDA. The Examples section includes an Archive of implementation guides from more than 40 projects worldwide.

21.5
Cross Enterprise Sharing of Medical Summaries (IHE)

At the same time that HL7 worked on the CRS, Integrating the Healthcare Enterprise was extending it to support CDA Level 3 entries in the newly created Patient Care Coordination Domain. The XDS-MS profile from IHE was to make use of the Care Record Summary, and produce level 3 structured entries for the most commonly needed data elements: Problems, Medications and Allergies.

This work was led in IHE by the author and by Dr. Dan Russler, one of the lead developers of the HL7 Care Record Draft Standard for Trial Use. It was greatly informed by the structures used for problems and allergies in that specification.

A few general principals were established early on in this implementation guide that has been carried forward by IHE and other organizations. Time intervals in HL7 can be represented in many different ways, but IHE specified that they would always be represented by using the <low> and <high> elements in an interval.

Narrative text would be referenced by the <text> element in the clinical statement act rather than duplicated to avoid a possible source of errors and to provide a link between clinical statements and the narrative text that they are associated with.

LOINC® would be used for Document Types and Sections (as recommended by HL7), and for laboratory results and test measurements.

The XDS-MS guide developed level 3 clinical statement specifications for problems, medications and allergies. That work subsequently informed the development of the HL7 Continuity of Care Document and later work in IHE on the ED Referral and Exchange of Personal Health Records specifications. It also influenced and was used in Health Story implementation guides that were balloted through HL7.

Subsequent work in IHE in the following year added just a couple of elements to the XDS-MS to support its used for ED referrals from a healthcare provider in the EDR profile.

The XDS-MS and EDR profiles can be found in the IHE Patient Care Coordination Technical Framework Volumes 1 and 2 on the IHE Website at: http://www.ihe.net/ Technical_Framework/index.cfm#pcc

21.6
The Continuity of Care Document

The HL7 Continuity of Care Document is perhaps the most widely known HL7 implementation guide in the world. Templates included in this specification are now included in more than 50 CDA implementation specifications developed by IHE, HL7, epSOS, the Chinese Ministry of Health, Continua, Health Story, AHIP and Blue Cross/Blue Shield, and numerous others.

This project emerged from the CRS/CCR debacle. After ASTM had finally prepared the CCR and published it, ASTM members began working in earnest with HL7 to produce a CDA guide that would support the CCR data set. The HL7 Structured Documents and Patient Care workgroups sponsored this work in HL7, but the CCD specification involved numerous clinical and administrative/financial domains from across the HL7 membership.

The Orders and Observations workgroup participated in the development of the CDA models that were used to report laboratory results in the CCD Results section. At nearly the same time, the IHE Laboratory domain was developing the XD-LAB profile, which would be a CDA profile for sharing laboratory results. They used that initial work as a springboard to develop that profile.

The HL7 Financial Management Workgroup participated in the development of the Payers section in the CCD. That work was based upon that workgroups model for representing patient insurance information.

The Clinical Genomics workgroup participated in the development of the Family History model. That model was the subject of much debate because the Clinical Genomics Pedigree standard could not be represented in the CDA using the same structures or relationships. An alternative model was used which allowed the information to be captured according to an analysis of the required domain information.

The concern class had been introduced into the HL7 RIM by the Patient Care Workgroup. This class was intended to represent an item of concern on a healthcare providers working list. This model also did not fit into the CDA Clinical Statement model directly, but we were able to resolve these issues by using the generic Act class to represent the concern act in CDA. This is why you see an act at the head of problem and allergy observations in the CCD today. The Concern act captures the clinically relevant information about when a healthcare provider became concerned about a problem reported by a patient.

The problems and allergies models developed by Patient Care were used to support recording of these times in the Conditions and Alerts section of the CCD.

The CCD specification is available free to HL7 members, and for a modest fee to non-members on the HL7 Website. You can find all HL7 CDA based standards and implementation guides at http://www.hl7.org/implement/standards/cda.cfm

21.7
Exchange of Personal Health Records

The Exchange of Personal Health Records profile, like the XDS-MS profile before it, was developed concurrently with the HL7 implementation guide that it was based upon. This guide sought to bring a degree of conformity between the HL7 CCD and the previous IHE XDS-MS profile, and to further constrain the CCD to support a specific use case of PHR exchange.

Because the CCD used the same requirements found in the ASTM CCR, a CCD document could contain as little as one section of data, and still be valid according to the business rules of the CCD. But for use in a healthcare environment, especially in exchanges with personal health record systems, IHE felt that there should be minimum requirements on the sections that were included.

In addition, the HL7 CCD guide still provided too many options in the way that problems could be reported. Problems could be reported in as many as three different ways, depending upon how you chose to do so. IHE felt that there should be only one way to accomplish this task, and that it should be done in a way that provided as much information as possible in the resulting document.

IHE required that the extract from the PHR or EHR that was being communicated contain at the very minimum, problems, medications, and allergies, as well as certain personal information for the patient. It also reused the general requirements of CRS on the CDA header, to ensure that all providers and the patient were identified.

Finally, it recommended that the content also include the patient preferred language, contacts, payers, the patient's pharmacy, advance directives, encounter history, and immunization history.

The IHE XPHR specification can be found in the IHE PCC Technical Framework Volume 2 on the IHE Website accessible from: http://www.ihe.net/Technical_Framework/index.cfm#pcc

21.8
The ANSI/HITSP C32 Summary Documents Using the CCD

At the same time that IHE was developing XPHR and HL7 was developing CCD, ANSI/HITSP was trying to solve the Consumer Empowerment use case in its first year. The use case delivered to ANSI/HITSP had included the CCR data elements almost verbatim. It took about six months of debate to determine how to proceed, because this was still a huge subject of debate in the healthcare standards space. Finally, the IHE XPHR profile was proposed as a solution for the use case, with HITSP to constrain vocabulary to support use in the US. Although the CCD was already US implementation guide. But because it followed the ASTM CCR requirements, it did not include US-centric vocabulary constraints which would have made the HITSP work unnecessary. This was in fact fortunate as it allowed the CCD to gain broad international support.

As one of the editors of both the CCD and the XPHR guides, I was also drafted to help develop the HITSP C32 specification by my colleague, Charles Parisot, who was one of the co-chairs of the Consumer Empowerment workgroup. The staff editor Don Van Syckle and I worked several very late nights to pull this specification together at the last minute.

That original draft was rejected in favor of using CCD directly. XPHR was viewed by some as being an invention of IHE that was competing with the ASTM and HL7 joint CCD development. Nothing could have been further from the truth. IHE had always intended that XPHR be conformant to the CCD specification and was working closely with HL7 to ensure this. While it took almost two weeks of effort to write the first draft (packed into three days by two people), changing the guide to make it depend upon CCD instead of XPHR was comparatively a rather small change.

ANSI/HITSP strongly supported the work of the HL7 CCD project, and even wrote an open letter strongly in support of it just before the final CCD ballot in December of 2006.

After about another year, ANSI/HITSP had developed a number of implementation guides which used IHE profiles, but still retained direct use of the CCD. This resulted in inconsistencies between the HITSP implementation guides where a problem section in one HITSP document could not be transferred to a problem section in another HITSP document without having to be modified. In early 2008 ANSI/HITSP began to address these difficulties, and by the end of that year, the IHE XPHR specification was incorporated back into the HITSP C32 specification.

The key features of the C32 introduced at that the time it was developed were principal that later developed into separate HITSP documents. The C32 was to be carried forward into the HITSP C83 CDA Sections and Entries, C80 Clinical Document and Message Terminology and C154 HITSP Data Dictionary later.

One of these features was the identification of the data elements that needed to be communicated. Each data element was given and identifier, a name, and a definition. The latter was absolutely critical, as it represented the agreed upon meaning for those short phrases that were given to HITSP in later use cases, and became the foundation for the HITSP C154 Data Dictionary. That document is very similar to what is produced during the early stages of an HL7 Domain Analysis process.

After the definitions, a table mapping each of the data elements was produced that showed how that data element was mapped into the selected standard. In this case, these were the HL7 CCD and CDA. XPath was chosen as the mapping language to explain where the data elements could be found.

Each mapped data element was also associated with a separate section in the original C32 specification which introduced further constraints and provided examples of how the CDA implementation should be produced. Those further constraints specified which vocabularies were allowed, or what identifiers should be used.

This information was later migrated in 2008 into a separate specification called the C83 CDA Content Modules Component, and merged with similarly created sections based on other HITSP specifications. The vocabulary constraints were also moved to a separate document called the C80 Clinical Document and Message Terminology Component.

The movement of this material out of the C32 and into the C83 and C80 specifications made it much easier for HITSP to manage consistency across its implementation guides. But it had the unfortunate side effect of requiring developers to "peel the onion", unwrapping layers of constraints before they could finally get all the details.

It was not uncommon for developers to need to refer to six different documents produced by three different organizations at the same time in order to implement a specification. This is a challenge that the Office of the National Coordinator in the US is presently attempting to address with the rather large and newly reconstituted US National Program known as the Standards and Interoperability Framework. One aspect of this challenge is that there needs to be a way to support the use of intellectual property from the many different organizations that provide supporting materials that are used. Another challenge that HITSP faced was the lack of appropriate tools or staff to support the quantity of work that it was asked to produce.

The original HITSP C32 document is still one of the best implementation guides I have ever worked on. You can find some of the earlier versions on the ANSI/HITSP website, which is still maintained by ANSI at http://www.hitsp.org. Version 2.1 of the HITSP C32 specification is still a "whole" specification. All of the HITSP guides mentioned above, and many others are freely available on that web site.

21.9
Laboratory Reports

At the same time HL7 was working on the CCD specification, the IHE Laboratory domain had used that work as a springboard to develop a CDA implementation guide for laboratory reports. This was certainly not the first such project, but it was the first such project to attempt to develop an International guide. Credit for the first project should probably go the Italian born guide: Specifiche tecniche per il referto di laboratorio secondo lo standard HL7 CDA Release 2.0.

The IHE Sharing Laboratory Reports profile was also being developed at the same time that ANSI/HITSP was trying to address the Laboratory Reporting use case (in the same year that the guides for the Consumer Empowerment use case were being developed). Members of IHE, ANSI/HITSP and HL7 followed this project around to meetings of all three organizations, and collaborated on its development.

The guide was finished later that year, and was subsequently adopted by ANSI/HITSP for use in the Laboratory Reporting use case in the C37 Lab Report Document component specification. Subsequently, when the HL7 Attachments workgroup revised the Laboratory Reporting guide, it produced a specification that built upon the HITSP and IHE work as well. It was designed so that if an implementer used the ANSI/HITSP specifications, all requirements of the Claims Attachments guide would be met. While it might have been easier to simply replace the existing HL7 Claims Attachment guide with the HITSP Guide from an overall effort perspective that would have been a huge hurdle for the Claims Attachment workgroup to overcome because of the different in styles used for the HITSP guide.

The HITSP C37 Laboratory Report Document is available from the HITSP website at http://www.hitsp.org.

The IHE Sharing Laboratory Reports specification is available in Volume 3 of the IHE Laboratory Technical Framework on the IHE website at: http://www.ihe.net/Technical_Framework/index.cfm#laboratory.

The draft of the HL7 Claims attachments implementation guides containing the CDA Release 2 Laboratory Implementation Specification balloted in HL7 May of 2007 can be found on the HL7 ballot site at: http://www.hl7.org/ctl.cfm?action=ballots.home&ballot_cycle_id=510. Please note that this is not the final publication.

21.10
Smart Open Services for European Patients

The epSOS project is an EU project that started with 12 EU member states. The goal of this project is to develop an EU framework that enables cross-border exchange of patient information. The first two CDA based specifications that this project developed were to support patient summaries and ePrescribing/eDispensation.

This project adopted a large number of the existing templates developed in the IHE PCC Technical Framework, and as a result was able to spend a good portion of their time addressing some of the more difficult challenges that this (or any project of similar scope) faced.

One of the challenges of this project was the lack of a common vocabulary for medications or a common regulatory structure or availability of medications. The problem this introduces in cross border case is one where a patient may be directed to take a particular drug in one country, but not be able to because it is not available in another country, and the pharmacist may also be challenged to find an appropriate substitute due to lack of knowledge about the original drugs constituents.

The epSOS project team solved this problem by using an existing HL7 model from the Medication domain as an extension to CDA. That extension allows the detailed components of the medication to be described so that the pharmacist can identify an appropriate substitute when necessary.

The epSOS CDA specifications can be found on the epSOS website at http://www. epsos.eu. The CDA guides can be downloaded from the web page describing Work Product D3.5.2 Semantic Services Specification.

21.11
Unstructured Documents

All of the implementation described above support at least level 2, if not level 3 structured content and entries. However, there are still many use cases for exchanging unstructured documentation. It is still in many cases the lowest common denominator between EHR systems, and also the quickest and easiest way to exchange clinical information.

IHE developed an implementation guide called Cross Enterprise Sharing of Scanned Documents, or XDS-SD that supports exchange of documents using the PDF/A standard, wrapped inside a CDA header. That specification can be found in Volume 3 of the IHE ITI Technical Framework at http://www.ihe.net/Technical_Framework/index.cfm#IT

ANSI/HITSP made use of that specification in its C62 Unstructured Documents component which can be found on the HITSP website at http://www.hitsp.org.

The Health Story project developed a similar guide as an HL7 DSTU addressing the needs of transcription systems and balloted it through the HL7 process. The HL7 Unstructured Document is designed as a superset of the IHE Scanned Document Specification, to meet the broader requirements of transcription products. All HL7 DSTUs can be found on the HL7 DSTU page at http://www.hl7.org/dstucomments/. Health Story developed specifications can also be found on the Health Story website at http://health-story.com/standards/standards.htm.

Summary

- There are more than 100 CDA implementation guides around the world.
- The first CDA Release 2.0 implementation guide was finished before the CDA Release 2.0 standard was complete.
- Most of the implementation guides can be located on the web and are freely accessible for anyone to read or use.

Questions

1. When was the first CDA Release 2.0 Implementation produced?
2. What technology did it introduce?
3. Which two HL7 implementation guides did IHE use for integration profiles at the same time as they were being produced by HL7?
4. What other organization worked on similar implementation guides at the same time as IHE was developing them?
5. Where can you find more than 40 implementation guides in one place?
6. Which implementation guides did not borrow from existing work?

Research Questions

1. Where would you find a collection of CDA Implementation Guides for Obstetric workflows? Emergency Care Workflows?
2. Which CDA Implementation guides are used in Programs in your region? How would you find out?*

Afterword

Once again I find myself awake in the early morning hours finishing up a CDA™ related project.

I have been deeply involved in the development of CDA Release 2.0 and the subsequent implementation guides developed by HL7, IHE, ANSI/HITSP and a few abroad for the last seven years. Over the course of those years I have learned a great deal about healthcare, standards, politics, sushi and sake. While this book is now finished, there is more to be done. I may shift my attention to other things, but CDA will always be very important to me. I expect to be involved in projects expanding upon CDA to support broader application. I also hope to see it simplified. The original title of this book was *The Little CDA™ Book*. This is not a little book, and even as large as it is, there are as many pages again more to tell. I hope in a few years that I can write a second edition that is half the size of this one. That will be an interesting challenge.

Healthcare Standards is not a career for me, rather it is a calling. I know that millions of people have accessible health records where they live because of some of the specifications that I have helped develop. What I truly want for myself and for my family is that we can have that where we live. There has been nothing more satisfying in my career than learning that the hospital I would use in an emergency uses standards and implementation guides that I have helped to develop.

I hope you will find the same sense of satisfaction and accomplishment in your careers. I also hope that you take what you learn from this book to the next step. I want to see a world where every patient can carry their health record around electronically, and where no care is delayed due to lack of information. For that to happen you need to take what have learned here and make it real where you live.

I also want to hear from you about your questions, your successes, and yes, your failures, or mine, either in this book or in the specifications that I helped to developed. It is only by communicating that we learn. You can reach me via the "Contact Me" link on my blog, which you can find on the web at http://motorcycleguy.blogspot.com.

Keith W. Boone

K.W. Boone, *The CDA™ Book*,
DOI: 10.1007/978-0-85729-336-7, © Springer-Verlag London Limited 2011

About the Author

Keith W. Boone has been involved in the development of Health Level 7 standards including the HL7 Clinical Document Architecture since 2004. He co-chaired the HL7 Structured Documents working group from 2007 to 2010, which is the home of CDA™ in Health Level 7 International. He is presently a member at large of the HL7 Board.

Keith also co-chairs the Integrating the Healthcare Enterprise (IHE) Patient Care Coordination (PCC) planning committee which develops CDA Implementation Guides (which IHE calls profiles) for use internationally. He co-chaired the technical committee of that group from 2006 to 2009.

He also co-chaired the ANSI/HITSP Care Management and Health Records (CMHR) domain technical committee which developed the ANSI/HITSP C32 Summary Documents using CCD and the ANSI/HITSP C83 CDA Document Content Module specifications, and the Data Architecture tiger team which developed the ANSI/HITSP C152 Data Dictionary specification.

He also participates in other standards organizations, including the US Technical Advisory Group to ISO TC-215, ASTM and Continua.

Mr. Boone is a Standards Architect for GE Healthcare, where he is currently employed, and represents GE Healthcare to numerous standard organizations. He was introduced to IHE profiles and HL7 standards while working as a Chief Engineer at Dictaphone Corporation where he took on the role of leading that organization's efforts in standards. Before he developed an interest in the HL7 Clinical Document Architecture, Keith was a Software Architect for eBusiness Technologies, an XML technology company. There he was introduced to standards development, and worked alongside many of the co-chairs and developers of the XML specifications, including XML, XML Namespaces, XSLT, and XPath.

Index

K.W. Boone, *The CDA Book*,
DOI: 10.1007/978-0-85729-336-7, © Springer-Verlag London Limited 2011

Printed by Publishers' Graphics LLC
CAMZ140309.20.06.18